CONCISE GUIDE TO
Anxiety Disorders

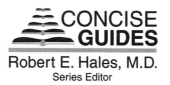

CONCISE GUIDES

Robert E. Hales, M.D.
Series Editor

CONCISE GUIDE TO
Anxiety Disorders

Eric Hollander, M.D.

Professor
Director of Clinical Psychopharmacology
Director, Compulsive, Impulsive and Anxiety Disorders Program
Department of Psychiatry
Mount Sinai School of Medicine, New York, New York

Daphne Simeon, M.D.

Associate Professor
Department of Psychiatry
Mount Sinai School of Medicine, New York, New York

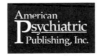

American Psychiatric Publishing, Inc.

Washington, DC
London, England

Copyright © 2003 American Psychiatric Publishing, Inc.
ALL RIGHTS RESERVED

Manufactured in the United States of America on acid-free paper
07 06 05 04 03   5 4 3 2 1
First Edition

American Psychiatric Publishing, Inc.
1400 K Street, N.W.
Washington, DC 20005
www.appi.org

Library of Congress Cataloging-in-Publication Data
Hollander, Eric, 1957-
    Concise guide to anxiety disorders / Eric Hollander, Daphne Simeon.
        p. ; cm.
    Includes bibliographical references and index.
    ISBN 1-58562-080-7 (alk. paper)
    1. Anxiety. I. Simeon, Daphne, 1958- II. Title.
    [DNLM: 1. Anxiety Disorders. WM 172 H737c 2002]
    RC531 .H655 2002
    616.85′223—dc21

                                                                        2002027684

British Library Cataloguing in Publication Data
A CIP record is available from the British Library.

CONTENTS

5 Psychological Theories...................125

LIST OF TABLES

3 Course and Prognosis

4 Biological Theories

5 Psychological Theories

6 Somatic Treatments

7 Psychotherapy Treatments

INTRODUCTION

to the Concise Guides Series

The Concise Guides Series from American Psychiatric Publishing, Inc., provides, in an accessible format, practical information for psychiatrists, psychiatry residents, and medical students working in a variety of treatment settings, such as inpatient psychiatry units, outpatient clinics, consultation-liaison services, and private office settings. The Concise Guides are meant to complement the more detailed information to be found in lengthier psychiatry texts.

The Concise Guides address topics of special concern to psychiatrists in clinical practice. The books in this series contain a detailed table of contents, along with an index, tables, figures, and other charts for easy access. The books are designed to fit into a lab coat pocket or jacket pocket, which makes them a convenient source of information. References have been limited to those most relevant to the material presented.

Robert E. Hales, M.D., M.B.A.
Series Editor, Concise Guides

PREFACE

Anxiety disorders are the most common of all psychiatric illnesses and result in considerable functional impairment and distress. Recent research developments have had a broad impact on our understanding of the underlying mechanisms of illness and treatment response. An explosion of research has led to dramatic developments in the understanding and alleviation of various forms of anxiety and has made the anxiety disorders an exciting field in modern psychiatry. Working with patients who have an anxiety disorder can be highly gratifying for the informed psychiatrist, because these patients, who are in considerable distress and often dysfunctional to varying degrees, frequently respond to proper treatment and achieve a higher level of functioning as well as life satisfaction. The major anxiety disorders covered in this guide are panic disorder, generalized anxiety disorder, social phobia, specific phobias, obsessive-compulsive disorder, and posttraumatic stress disorder. We have endeavored to present comprehensive summaries of epidemiology and comorbidity, diagnosis and differential diagnosis, biological and psychological theories, and finally treatment by medication, psychotherapy, or combined approaches. We have aimed to make each chapter concise and reader-friendly and at the same time thorough in its scope and latest referencing.

ACKNOWLEDGMENTS

We thank Dorothy Nelson, B.S., for her assistance on this project.

EPIDEMIOLOGY

Highlights from the epidemiology of anxiety disorders, including prevalence, sex ratio, and comorbidity, are summarized in Table 1–1.

■ PANIC DISORDER

The anxiety disorders have all been included in our large national epidemiologic studies of mental illness during the years 1982–2002, and we can therefore be fairly confident about prevalence estimates of anxiety disorders in the general United States population. In an early study, the National Institute of Mental Health Epidemiologic Catchment Area (ECA) study, researchers examined the population prevalence of anxiety disorders at five sites, based on DSM-III (American Psychiatric Association 1980) criteria and using the Diagnostic Interview Schedule (DIS) (Regier et al. 1988). The 1-month, 6-month, and lifetime prevalence rates for panic disorder were 0.5%, 0.8%, and 1.6%, respectively. Women had a 1-month prevalence rate of 0.7%, which was significantly higher than the 0.3% rate found among men; women also tended to have a greater rise in panic disorder at ages 25–44 years, and their attacks tended to continue longer into older age (Regier et al. 1988). More recent epidemiologic study using the DSM-III-R (American Psychiatric Association 1987) criteria found a lifetime prevalence of 3.5% and 1-year prevalence of 2.3% for panic disorder (Kessler et al. 1994). Again, women were more than twice as likely to have had lifetime panic disorder (5%) than men (2%).

The relationship between panic disorder and major depression has been examined in numerous studies, because the two are well

TABLE 1–1. Approximate lifetime prevalence, gender ratio, and common comorbidities for the major anxiety disorders

Disorder	Prevalence (%)	Females:males	Comorbidity
Panic disorder	2–4	> 2:1	Depression, other anxiety disorders
GAD	5–7	2:1	Overall 90%; 50%–60% for major depression or other anxiety disorder
Social phobia	13–16	> 1:1	2-fold risk for alcohol dependence; 3- to 6-fold risk of mood disorders
Specific phobias	10	2:1	Depression and somatoform
Agoraphobia	6	2:1	Not well established
OCD	2–3	1:1	Anxiety, depression, tics, hypochondriasis, eating disorder, body dysmorphic disorder (childhood-onset more common in males)
PTSD	7–9	2:1	Depression, OCD, panic, phobias

Note. GAD = generalized anxiety disorder; OCD = obsessive-compulsive disorder; PTSD = posttraumatic stress disorder.

known to commonly co-occur. A recent family study found that panic disorder and major depression are clearly distinct disorders—despite their substantial co-occurrence—and panic comorbid with major depression does not segregate in families as a distinct disorder (Weissman et al. 1993).

It has not been clearly established whether particular personality types are correlated with panic disorder, and studies are further confounded because the presence of panic disorder may have secondary effects on personality. Noyes et al. (1991) conducted personality follow-ups of panic disorder patients who had been treated for panic for 3 years and found that the initial avoidant and dependent traits were to a large extent related to panic and waned with its treatment. On the other hand, experience leads many clinicians to feel that patients with agoraphobia and panic are more likely to have histories of dependent character traits that antedate the onset of panic. This association is a difficult subject to study, because the research would require a longitudinal design assessing personality before the onset of Axis I disorders as a baseline; consequently, we do not have definitive answers.

■ GENERALIZED ANXIETY DISORDER

Generalized anxiety disorder (GAD) findings from the ECA study must be interpreted with caution, because this disorder was assessed only in the second wave of the study, and only at three of the five sites. Also, the DIS criteria that were used to make the diagnosis, in accordance with DSM-III, required a total of only three somatic symptoms and only a 1-month duration of illness and therefore could be an overestimate according to current criteria. One-year prevalence rates for the three sites combined were 3.8% without any exclusions, 2.7% when concurrent panic or major depression was excluded, and 1.7% when any other DSM-III diagnoses were excluded. Lifetime prevalence when panic and major depression were excluded ranged from 4.1% to 6.6%, depending on the site. Rates were higher overall in women (Blazer et al. 1991).

Another large epidemiologic study, the National Comorbidity Survey (NCS), assessed DSM-III-R GAD and found that it had a current (past year) prevalence of 3.1% and a lifetime prevalence of 5.1% in people ages 15–45 years, was twice as common in women, and had a very high lifetime comorbidity of 90% with a wide spectrum of other psychiatric disorders (Kessler et al. 1994). Even so, the prevalence and comorbidity patterns of current GAD supported its conceptualization as a distinct disorder (Wittchen et al. 1994). More recent studies following DSM-IV (American Psychiatric Association 1994) criteria (Carter et al. 2001) have confirmed a similar epidemiology for GAD, with a one-year prevalence of 1.5% for threshold GAD and 3.6% for subthreshold GAD. Higher rates of the disorder were found in women (2.7%) and in elderly people (2.2%). A high degree of comorbidity was again confirmed: 59% for major depression and 56% for other anxiety disorders.

Despite its high comorbidity with other anxiety disorders and with mood disorders, it has become increasingly evident in recent years that GAD stands on its own as a disorder with distinct onset, course, impairment, and prognosis. Epidemiologic data have revealed that GAD and depression each show their own statistically significant and independent associations with impairment—of roughly equal magnitude—which cannot be accounted for by comorbidity or sociodemographic variables (Kessler et al. 1999a). On certain quality-of-life indexes, individuals with pure GAD actually fare worse than those with pure major depression (Wittchen et al. 2000).

With regard to Axis II comorbidity, the personality types of patients with GAD have not been well characterized. One study reported that approximately one-third of patients with GAD also had a DSM-III personality disorder, and the most common one was dependent personality disorder (Noyes et al. 1987). Avoidant personality disorder may also be common in GAD (Mavissakalian et al. 1993). However, as with panic disorder, it remains unclear whether such personality disorders are primary or consequent to the GAD itself. High levels of mistrust and anger have also been reported in GAD (Mavissakalian et al. 1993).

■ SPECIFIC PHOBIAS AND AGORAPHOBIA

In the ECA study, phobias as a group were found to be the most common current psychiatric disorder, with 1-month and 6-month prevalence rates of about 6% and 8%, respectively, and a lifetime rate of 12.5% (Regier et al. 1988). Specific phobias were the most common (11.3% lifetime prevalence), followed by agoraphobia (5.6%) and social phobia (2.7%). Median ages at illness onset were 15 years for specific phobias, 16 years for social phobia, and 29 years for agoraphobia. The phobias were highly comorbid with each other, and despite significant functional impairment, only a minority of the individuals interviewed had sought professional help.

In the more recent NCS (Kessler et al. 1994; Magee et al. 1996), which employed DSM-III-R criteria, specific phobias had the same lifetime prevalence (11.3%) as in the ECA study. Specific phobias were more common in women than in men (14.5% vs. 7.8%). In a community study of adolescents, the prevalence of specific phobias was found to be 3.5% higher in girls than in boys; there was also notable comorbidity with depressive and somatoform disorders in about one-third of the sample (Essau et al. 2000). Most commonly, individuals never seek treatment for this disorder.

Agoraphobia in the NCS (Kessler et al. 1994) was similar to findings in the ECA study, with a lifetime prevalence of 6.7% and a 1-month prevalence of 2.3%; agoraphobia was more common in women (7.9%) than in men (3.2%). Agoraphobia in the absence of panic disorder is traditionally believed to be rare; therefore, for the purposes of this volume agoraphobia is discussed under panic disorder. Agoraphobia without any history of panic attacks is only infrequently encountered in clinical settings, a finding on which most studies and clinicians agree. Indeed, some investigators believe that an initial panic attack, even if remote or forgotten, is a necessary prerequisite for the development of agoraphobia. This conclusion is, however, controversial. For example, in one clinical series studying patients who had panic disorder with agoraphobia, 23% of patients reported that agoraphobia preceded the initial panic attack, although retrospective biases may cast some doubt on such a finding (Lelliott et al. 1989). Most striking is the high prevalence of agoraphobia without panic that has been reported in epidemiologic samples. The findings of the ECA study were that the majority of new-onset agoraphobia (about two-thirds) occurred without a history of panic attacks (Eaton and Keyl 1990). Such a discrepant finding may, at least in part, be accounted for by an excessively low severity threshold and weaknesses in differential diagnosis in epidemiologic assessments.

■ SOCIAL PHOBIA

The earliest epidemiologic study (ECA) found low prevalence of social phobia, a 2.8% lifetime prevalence rate (Schneier et al. 1992). However, the assessment of social phobia was incomplete, and this rate turned out to be a gross underestimate. Subsequently, the NCS identified a 13.3% lifetime and 7.9% 1-year prevalence (Magee et al. 1996). Of those individuals, about one-third reported exclusively public speaking fears, one-third had at least one additional social fear, and one-third had multiple fears qualifying for the generalized type of social phobia. Generalized social phobia was found to be more persistent, impairing, and comorbid than the specific public speaking type. However, the two types did not differ in age at onset, family history, and certain sociodemographic variables (Kessler et al. 1998). In a large epidemiologic survey of social phobia, Schneier et al. (1992) found that 70% of persons with social phobia were women. Mean age at onset was 15 years, and there was substantial associated morbidity, including greater financial dependency and greater suicidal ideation than in individuals without social phobia. Similarly, in a population-based adolescent female twin sample, the lifetime prevalence of social phobia was found to be 16% (Nelson et al. 2000), and those with social phobia already carried a threefold higher risk of comorbid major depression and a twofold higher risk of alcohol dependence. Social phobia with comorbid depression was associated with an elevated risk of alcohol problems and suicidality. Epidemiologic studies have consistently found significant comorbidity between lifetime social phobia and various mood disorders, with an approximately three- to sixfold higher risk for dysthymia, depression, and bipolar disorder (Kessler et al. 1999b). Almost always, social phobia predates the mood disorder and is a predictor not only of higher likelihood, but also of greater severity and chronicity, of future mood disorder.

Parental social phobia is a strong risk factor for social phobia among adolescent offspring, as is parental depression, any other anxiety disorder, any alcohol use disorder, and parental overprotection or rejection, whereas overall family functioning is not predictive (Lieb et al. 2000). Other risk factors for social phobia identified in a large epidemiologic sample include lack of a close relationship with an adult, not being firstborn for males, parental marital conflict, parental history of psychiatric disorder, moving several times as a child, childhood abuse, running away from home, and doing poorly in school (Chartier et al. 2001). These variables remained largely significant when controlling for comorbidity. Risk factors for developing social phobia are summarized in Table 1–2.

TABLE 1–2.   Risk factors for social phobia

Parental psychiatric history (especially social phobia, other anxiety disorders, depression)

Parental marital conflict

Parental overprotection or rejection

Childhood abuse

Childhood lack of close relationship with an adult

Not being first-born for males

Frequent moves in childhood

Poor school performance

Running away from home

Social phobia can be associated with a variety of personality disorders, and in particular avoidant personality disorder (Dyck et al. 2001). In epidemiologically identified probands with social phobia alone, avoidant personality disorder alone, or both, there has been found a similarly elevated familial risk of social phobia, suggesting that the Axis I and Axis II disorders may represent dimensions of social anxiety rather than discrete conditions (Tillfors et al. 2001). Indeed, in a recent review of the literature comparing generalized social phobia, avoidant personality disorder, and shyness, researchers concluded that all three may exist on a continuum (Rettew 2000).

Social phobia, in and of itself, is a highly disabling disorder, whose impact on functioning and quality of life has probably been greatly underestimated and hidden in past years. Recent studies (Stein and Kean 2000) show that persons with social phobia are impaired on a broad spectrum of measures, ranging from dropping out of school to significant disability in whatever is their main activity. People with social phobia describe dissatisfaction with many aspects of their life, and the quality of their life is rated as quite low. Importantly, comorbid depression seems to contribute only modestly to these outcomes. Even in preadolescent children, pervasive and serious functional impairment can already be found (Beidel et al. 1999).

■ OBSESSIVE-COMPULSIVE DISORDER

Obsessive-compulsive disorder (OCD) used to be considered one of the rarest mental disorders, and early studies suggested a maximum incidence of 5 in 10,000 persons (Woodruff and Pitts 1964). This low figure was probably due to clinicians' unfamiliarity with the disorder until the 1990s, OCD patients' secretiveness about their symptoms, and an average wait of 7.5 years before patients seek psychiatric help (Rasmussen and Tsuang 1986). However, data from the ECA study first documented that OCD is a fairly common mental disorder, with a 1-month prevalence of 1.3%, a 6-month prevalence of 1.5%, and a lifetime rate of 2.5% (Regier et al. 1988).

In clinical samples of adult OCD, there is a roughly equal ratio of men to women (Black 1974). The ECA sample found a slightly higher 1-month prevalence for women (1.5%) compared with men

(1.1%) that was accounted for in ages 25–64, but this difference is not significant (Karno et al. 1988; Regier et al. 1988). However, in childhood-onset OCD, about 70% of patients are male (Hollingsworth et al. 1980; Swedo et al. 1989). This difference seems to be accounted for by the earlier age at onset in males, and it may suggest partly differing etiologies or vulnerabilities in the two sexes.

There are reports demonstrating comorbidity of OCD with schizophrenia, depressive disorder or mood disorder, other anxiety disorders such as panic disorder and simple and social phobia, eating disorders, autistic disorder, Tourette syndrome, and other disorders in the obsessive-compulsive spectrum. Epidemiologically, the OCD comorbidity risk for other major psychiatric disorders was found to be fairly high but nondistinct (Karno et al. 1988). In a clinical sample of patients with schizophrenia and schizoaffective disorder, about 8% met criteria for OCD, highlighting the importance of screening for obsessive-compulsive symptoms in such populations, in which detection may be more difficult (Eisen et al. 1997).

What about Axis II comorbidity in OCD? Traditional psychoanalytic theorists suggest that there is a continuum between compulsive personality and OCD. Janet (1908) stated that all obsessional patients have a premorbid personality that is causally related to the disorder. Freud (1913/1958) noted an association between obsessional neurosis (i.e., OCD) symptoms and personality traits such as obstinacy, parsimony, punctuality, and orderliness. However, phenomenologic and epidemiologic evidence suggests that OCD is frequently distinct from obsessive-compulsive personality disorder. OCD symptoms are ego-dystonic, whereas obsessive-compulsive personality traits are ego-systonic and do not involve a sense of compulsion that must be resisted. Epidemiologic studies show that obsessive-compulsive character pathology is neither necessary nor sufficient for the development of OCD symptoms. When patients with obsessional traits decompensate, they often develop depression, paranoia, or somatization rather than OCD. Although the older literature suggested the presence of definite obsessional traits in as many as two-thirds of OCD patients, structured personality assessments were not used in evaluation. In more recent standardized evaluations, only a minority of OCD patients had DSM-III-R obsessive-compulsive personality disorder, whereas other personality disorders such as avoidant or dependent personality disorder were more common (Thomsen and Mikkelsen 1993). In addition, personality disorders might be more common in the presence of a longer duration of OCD—suggesting they could be secondary to the Axis I disorder—and criteria for personality disorders might no longer be met after successful treatment of the OCD (Baer et al. 1990; Baer and Jenike 1992). An interesting recent study suggests that there may exist a familial spectrum of obsessive-compulsive disorder and obsessive-compulsive personality disorder (Bienvenu et al. 2000).

■ POSTTRAUMATIC STRESS DISORDER

Although there are marked individual differences in how people react to stress, the rate of psychiatric morbidity starts to increase rapidly when stressors become extreme (Eitinger 1971; Krystal 1968). Although this disorder has been more extensively studied in select groups—such as survivors of combat, concentration camps, and natural disasters—researchers in the ECA study investigated the occurrence of PTSD in the general population (Helzer et al. 1987). A 1% lifetime prevalence of PTSD was found (0.5% in men and 1.3% in women). The nature of the precipitating trauma differed in the two sexes. Combat and witnessing someone's injury or death were the precipitating traumas identified in men, whereas physical attack or threat accounted for almost half of the traumas in women. In another large, random community survey of young adults, the lifetime prevalence of PTSD was 9.2%, higher than that of the ECA study (Breslau et al. 1991). As in the ECA study, the prevalence was higher in women (11.3%) than in men (6%). In the more recent NCS, the lifetime prevalence of PTSD was similarly found to be 7.8%, much higher than in the ECA study, and was more common in women. The most common stressors were combat exposure in men and sexual assault in women (Kessler et al. 1995).

Symptoms of PTSD too few in number to meet the full diagnostic criteria are quite common in the general population. In a Canadian community survey, full PTSD was found in 2.7% of women and 1.2% of men, and partial PTSD was found in an additional 3.4% of women and 0.3% of men. Individuals with partial PTSD, seemingly women in particular, may be important to identify, because they can be experiencing clinically meaningful distress and functional impairment (Stein et al. 1997). The gender difference in PTSD prevalence, higher in women, has been consistent across a number of studies. It appears that women are more likely to develop PTSD than men with comparable exposure to traumatic events, especially if exposure is before age 15 (Breslau et al. 1997). This difference is not well understood and could involve characteristics of both the individuals and the traumatic experiences.

A high rate of comorbid disorders is found in PTSD. In the ECA study, the rate of comorbidity was highest with affective disorders and OCD. Men with PTSD had no increased risk for panic disorder or phobias, whereas women with PTSD had a three- to fourfold risk of these disorders (Helzer et al. 1987). In the survey conducted by Breslau and colleagues (1991), a high rate of comorbidity was found for OCD, agoraphobia, panic, and depression, whereas the association with drug or alcohol abuse was weaker. The comorbidity of PTSD with depression is a very consistent one, and the nature of the relationship between the two conditions is controversial. Epidemiologic analyses suggest that among persons exposed to traumatic events the vulnerabilities for PTSD and depression are not separate; rather, the risk for depression is highly elevated in just those who manifest PTSD (Breslau et al. 2000). On the other hand, a prospective study of a large sample of trauma survivors found depression and PTSD to be independent sequelae of trauma (Shalev et al. 1998a). Regardless of causality, it is clear that PTSD in women increases the risk for new onset of both depression and alcohol use disorder (Breslau et al. 1997). Individuals with PTSD may be more likely to manifest borderline or self-defeating personality disorder and, interestingly, it appears that the actual PTSD diagnosis rather than the trauma history may account for this association (Shea et al. 2000).

There is general agreement in the literature that a variety of pre-morbid risk factors predispose to the development of PTSD (see Table 1–3). Although the disorder can certainly develop in people without significant preexisting psychopathology, a number of biological and psychological variables have been identified that render individuals more vulnerable to the development of PTSD. In one study of a Vietnam veteran outreach center, a prior history of good adolescent friendships was predictive of PTSD, whereas a history of poor adolescent friendships was more likely in those who did not have PTSD. In addition, this study reported a number of patients with good premorbid adjustment, low childhood trauma, and good adolescent relationships who experienced prolonged trauma in Vietnam and developed severe PTSD (Lindy et al. 1984). In general, however, previous adversity has been associated with a higher likelihood of developing PTSD.

For a long time it has been suggested that the greater the amount of previous trauma experienced by an individual, the more likely he or she is to develop symptoms after a stressful life event (Horowitz et al. 1980). Data that have been generated starting in the 1980s confirm how true this is. In addition, individuals with prior traumatic experiences may be more likely to become exposed to future traumas, because they can be prone to behaviorally reenact the original trauma (van der Kolk 1989). In a study of Vietnam veterans, those with PTSD had higher rates of childhood physical abuse than those without PTSD, as well as a considerably higher rate of total traumatic events prior to joining the military (Bremner et al. 1993).

TABLE 1–3.   **Risk factors for PTSD**

Past history of trauma prior to the index trauma
Past history of PTSD
Past history of depression
Past history of anxiety disorders
Comorbid Axis II disorders (predictive of greater chronicity)
Family history of anxiety (including parental PTSD)
Disrupted parental attachments
Severity of exposure to trauma (more predictive of acute symptoms)

Note.   PTSD = posttraumatic stress disorder.

McFarlane (1989) found that the severity of exposure to disaster was the major determinant of early posttraumatic morbidity, whereas preexisting psychological disorders better predicted the persistence of posttraumatic symptoms over time. A number of psychiatric conditions in probands and in their relatives appear to predispose individuals toward developing PTSD. In the ECA sample, a history of childhood conduct problems before age 15 was predictive of PTSD. Patients with anxious premorbid states and family histories of anxiety may also respond to a trauma with pathological anxiety and develop PTSD (Scrignar 1984). An epidemiologic survey identified, albeit retrospectively, different risk factors for becoming exposed to trauma versus developing PTSD following traumatic exposure (Breslau et al. 1991). Risk factors for exposure to trauma were male sex, childhood conduct problems, extraversion, and family history of substance abuse or psychiatric problems. Risk factors for developing PTSD after traumatic exposure included disrupted parent-child attachments, anxiety, depression, and family history of anxiety. Having an Axis II disorder also increases the risk for chronic PTSD (Ursano et al. 1999a). Having a past history of PTSD increases the risk for both acute and chronic PTSD (Ursano et al. 1999a). Compared with nonchronic PTSD, chronic PTSD of greater than 1 year's duration has been specifically associated with higher rates of comorbid anxiety and depressive disorders and a family history of antisocial behavior (Breslau and Davis 1992). Interestingly, parental PTSD is also a risk factor for PTSD in offspring, even in the absence of elevated trauma (Yehuda et al. 1998a). Findings with regard to gender are conflicting, in that female gender has been associated with chronic PTSD in one study (Breslau and Davis 1992) but only with acute PTSD in another (Ursano et al. 1999a). An additional risk factor that has been associated with higher likelihood of developing PTSD is lower premorbid intelligence (Macklin et al. 1998). Neurologic compromise, with increased neurologic soft signs and childhood histories of neurodevelopmental problems and lower intelligence, is associated with PTSD and could possibly be a predisposing risk factor (Gurvits et al. 2000).

Early predictors of PTSD after a traumatic event have also received great attention, and their potential significance for early intervention and prevention is obvious. As previously stated, the occurrence of acute stress disorder in the first month after trauma is a very strong predictor of later PTSD. Acute stress disorder diagnosis combined with a resting heart rate greater than 90 beats/minute has a surprisingly high sensitivity (88%) and specificity (85%) in predicting development of PTSD (Bryant et al. 2000). Similarly, high heart rate and decreased cortisol levels in the acute aftermath of trauma strongly correlate with later PTSD (Yehuda et al. 1998b). Even elevated heart rate alone, shortly after trauma, is a strong predictor of later PTSD (Shalev et al. 1998b). The importance of the very early reaction to a traumatic event in predicting PTSD should not be underestimated. Early PTSD-type symptoms within 1 week of a traffic accident predict the occurrence of PTSD as much as 1 year later (Koren et al. 1999).

Increased attention in recent years to dissociative phenomena and to their relationship to posttraumatic symptoms reveals that greater dissociation around the time of the traumatic event also is a strong predictor of the later development of PTSD (Marmar et al. 1994; Shalev et al. 1996). Individuals with peritraumatic dissociation are four to five times more likely to develop both acute and chronic PTSD (Ursano et al. 1999b). It may be that early peritraumatic dissociation can serve as a "marker" to identify individuals who will be at high risk of developing future PTSD.

■ REFERENCES

American Psychiatric Association: Diagnostic and Statistical Manual of Mental Disorders, 3rd Edition. Washington, DC, American Psychiatric Association, 1980

American Psychiatric Association: Diagnostic and Statistical Manual of Mental Disorders, 3rd Edition, Revised. Washington, DC, American Psychiatric Association, 1987

American Psychiatric Association: Diagnostic and Statistical Manual of Mental Disorders, 4th Edition. Washington, DC, American Psychiatric Association, 1994

Baer L, Jenike MA: Personality disorders in obsessive-compulsive disorder. Psychiatr Clin North Am 15:803–812, 1992

Baer L, Jenike MA, Ricciardi JN, et al: Standardized assessment of personality disorders in obsessive-compulsive disorder. Arch Gen Psychiatry 47:826–830, 1990

Beidel DC, Turner SM, Morris TL: Psychopathology of childhood social phobia. J Am Acad Child Adolesc Psychiatry 38:643–650, 1999

Bienvenu OJ, Samuels JF, Riddle MA, et al: The relationship of obsessive-compulsive disorder to possible spectrum disorders: results from a family study. Biol Psychiatry 48:287–293, 2000

Black A: The natural history of obsessional neurosis, in Obsessional States. Edited by Beech HK. London, Methuen Press, 1974, pp 19–54

Blazer DG, Hughes D, George LK: Generalized anxiety disorder, in Psychiatric Disorders in America. Edited by Robins LN, Regier DA. New York, Free Press, 1991, pp 180–203

Bremner JD, Southwick SM, Johnson DR, et al: Childhood physical abuse and combat-related posttraumatic stress disorder in Vietnam veterans. Am J Psychiatry 150:235–239, 1993

Breslau N, Davis GC: Posttraumatic stress disorder in an urban population of young adults: risk factors for chronicity. Am J Psychiatry 149:671–675, 1992

Breslau N, Davis GC, Andreski P, et al: Traumatic events and posttraumatic stress disorder in an urban population of young adults. Arch Gen Psychiatry 48:216–222, 1991

Breslau N, Davis GC, Andreski P, et al: Sex differences in posttraumatic stress disorder. Arch Gen Psychiatry 54:1044–1048, 1997

Breslau N, Davis GC, Peterson EL, et al: A second look at comorbidity in victims of trauma: the posttraumatic stress disorder-major depression connection. Biol Psychiatry 48:902–909, 2000

Bryant RA, Harvey AG, Guthrie RM, et al: A prospective study of psychophysiological arousal, acute stress disorder, and posttraumatic stress disorder. J Abnorm Psychol 109:341–344, 2000

Carter RM, Wittchen HU, Pfister H, et al: One-year prevalence of sub-threshold and threshold DSM-IV generalized anxiety disorder in a nationally representative sample. Depress Anxiety 13:78–88, 2001

Chartier MJ, Walker JR, Stein MB: Social phobia and potential childhood risk factors in a community sample. Psychol Med 31:307–315, 2001

Dyck IR, Phillips KA, Warshaw MG, et al: Patterns of personality pathology in patients with generalized anxiety disorder, panic disorder with and without agoraphobia, and social phobia. J Personal Disord 15:60–71, 2001

Eaton WW, Keyl PM: Risk factors for the onset of Diagnostic Interview Schedule/DSM-III agoraphobia in a prospective, population-based study. Arch Gen Psychiatry 47:819–824, 1990

Eisen JL, Beer DA, Pato MT, et al: Obsessive-compulsive disorder in patients with schizophrenia or schizoaffective disorder. Am J Psychiatry 154:271–273, 1997

Eitinger L: Organic and psychosomatic aftereffects of concentration camp imprisonment. Int Psychiatry Clin 8:205–215, 1971

Essau CA, Conradt J, Petermann F: Frequency, comorbidity, and psychosocial impairment of specific phobia in adolescents. J Clin Child Psychol 29:221–231, 2000

Freud S: The disposition to obsessional neurosis: A contribution to the problem of choice of neurosis (1913), in The Standard Edition of the Complete Psychological Works of Sigmund Freud, Vol 12. Translated and edited by Strachey J. London, Hogarth Press, 1958, pp 311–326

Gurvits TV, Gilbertson MW, Lasko NB, et al: Neurologic soft signs in chronic posttraumatic stress disorder. Arch Gen Psychiatry 57:181–186, 2000

Helzer JE, Robins LN, McEvoy L: Post-traumatic stress disorder in the general population: findings of the Epidemiologic Catchment Area survey. N Engl J Med 317:1630–1634, 1987

Hollingsworth CE, Tanguay PE, Grossman L, et al: Long-term outcome of obsessive-compulsive disorder in childhood. J Am Acad Child Psychiatry 19:134–144, 1980

Horowitz MJ, Wilner N, Kaltreider N, et al: Signs and symptoms of posttraumatic stress disorders. Arch Gen Psychiatry 37:88–92, 1980

Janet P: Les Obsessions et la Psychasthénie, 2nd Edition. Paris, Bailliere, 1908

Karno M, Golding JM, Sorenson SB, et al: The epidemiology of obsessive-compulsive disorder in five US communities. Arch Gen Psychiatry 45:1094–1099, 1988

Kessler RC, McGonagle KA, Zhao S, et al: Lifetime and 12-month prevalence of DSM-III-R psychiatric disorders in the United States; results from the National Comorbidity Survey. Arch Gen Psychiatry 51:8–19, 1994

Kessler RC, Sonnega A, Bromet E, et al: Posttraumatic stress disorder in the National Comorbidity Survey. Arch Gen Psychiatry 52:1048–1060, 1995

Kessler RC, Stein MB, Berglund P: Social phobia subtypes in the National Comorbidity Survey. Am J Psychiatry 155:613–619, 1998

Kessler RC, DuPont RL, Berglund P, et al: Impairment in pure and comorbid generalized anxiety disorder and major depression at 12 months in two national surveys. Am J Psychiatry 156:1915–1923, 1999a

Kessler RC, Stang P, Wittchen HU, et al: Lifetime co-morbidities between social phobia and mood disorders in the US National Comorbidity Survey. Psychol Med 29:555–567, 1999b

Koren D, Arnon I, Klein E: Acute stress response and posttraumatic stress disorder in traffic accident victims: a one-year prospective, follow-up study. Am J Psychiatry 156:367–373, 1999

Krystal H: Massive Psychic Trauma. New York, International Universities Press, 1968

Lelliott P, Marks I, McNamee G, et al: Onset of panic disorder with agoraphobia: toward an integrated model. Arch Gen Psychiatry 46:1000–1004, 1989

Lieb R, Wittchen HU, Hofler M, et al: Parental psychopathology, parenting styles, and the risk of social phobia in offspring: a prospective-longitudinal community study. Arch Gen Psychiatry 57:859–866, 2000

Lindy JD, Grace MC, Green BL: Building a conceptual bridge between civilian trauma and war trauma: preliminary psychological findings from a clinical sample of Vietnam veterans, in Post-Traumatic Stress Disorder: Psychological and Biological Sequelae. Edited by van der Kolk BA. Washington, DC, American Psychiatric Press, 1984, pp 44–57

Macklin ML, Metzger LJ, Litz BT, et al: Lower precombat intelligence is a risk factor for posttraumatic stress disorder. J Consult Clin Psychol 66:323–326, 1998

Magee WJ, Eaton WW, Wittchen HU, et al: Agoraphobia, simple phobia, and social phobia in the National Comorbidity Survey. Arch Gen Psychiatry 53:159–68, 1996

Marmar CR, Weiss DS, Schlenger WE, et al: Peritraumatic dissociation and posttraumatic stress in male Vietnam theater veterans. Am J Psychiatry 151:902–907, 1994

Mavissakalian M, Hamann MS, Haidar SA, et al: DSM-III personality disorders in generalized anxiety, panic/agoraphobia, and obsessive-compulsive disorders. Compr Psychiatry 34:243–248, 1993

McFarlane AC: The etiology of post-traumatic morbidity: predisposing, precipitating and perpetuating factors. Br J Psychiatry 154:221–228, 1989

Nelson EC, Grant JD, Bucholz KK, et al: Social phobia in a population-based female adolescent twin sample: co-morbidity and associated suicide-related symptoms. Psychol Med 30:797–804, 2000

Noyes R Jr, Clarkson C, Crow RR, et al: A family study of generalized anxiety disorder. Am J Psychiatry 144:1019–1024, 1987

Noyes R Jr, Reich JH, Suelzer M, et al: Personality traits associated with panic disorder: change associated with treatment. Compr Psychiatry 32:283–294, 1991

Rasmussen SA, Tsuang MT: Clinical characteristics and family history in DSM-III obsessive compulsive disorder. Am J Psychiatry 143:317–322, 1986

Regier DA, Boyd JH, Burke JD Jr, et al: One-month prevalence of mental disorders in the United States, based on five Epidemiologic Catchment Area sites. Arch Gen Psychiatry 45:977–986, 1988

Rettew DC: Avoidant personality disorder, generalized social phobia, and shyness: putting the personality back into personality disorders. Harv Rev Psychiatry 8:283–297, 2000

Schneier FR, Johnson J, Hornig CD, et al: Social phobia: comorbidity and morbidity in an epidemiologic sample. Arch Gen Psychiatry 49:282–288, 1992

Scrignar CB: Post-Traumatic Stress Disorder: Diagnosis, Treatment, and Legal Issues. New York, Praeger, 1984

Shalev AY, Peri T, Canetti L, et al: Predictors of PTSD in injured trauma survivors: a prospective study. Am J Psychiatry 153:2219–2225, 1996

Shalev AY, Freedman S, Peri T, et al: Prospective study of posttraumatic stress disorder and depression following trauma. Am J Psychiatry 155:630–637, 1998a

Shalev AY, Sahar T, Freedman S, et al: A prospective study of heart rate response following trauma and the subsequent development of posttraumatic stress disorder. Arch Gen Psychiatry 55:553–559, 1998b

Shea MT, Zlotnick C, Dolan R, et al: Personality disorders, history of trauma, and posttraumatic stress disorder in subjects with anxiety disorders. Compr Psychiatry 41:312–325, 2000

Stein MB, Kean YM: Disability and quality of life in social phobia: epidemiologic findings. Am J Psychiatry 157:1606–1613, 2000

Stein MB, Walker JR, Hazen AL, et al: Full and partial posttraumatic stress disorder: findings from a community survey. Am J Psychiatry 154:1114–1119, 1997

Swedo SE, Rapoport JL, Leonard H, et al: Obsessive-compulsive disorder in children and adolescents: clinical phenomenology of 70 consecutive cases. Arch Gen Psychiatry 46:335–341, 1989

Thomsen PH, Mikkelsen HU: Development of personality disorders in children and adolescents with obsessive-compulsive disorder: a 6- to 22-year follow-up study. Acta Psychiatr Scand 87:456–462, 1993

Tillfors M, Furmark T, Ekselius L, et al: Social phobia and avoidant personality disorder as related to parental history of social anxiety: a general population study. Behav Res Ther 39:289–298, 2001

Ursano RJ, Fullerton CS, Epstein RS, et al: Peritraumatic dissociation and posttraumatic stress disorder following motor vehicle accidents. Am J Psychiatry 156:1808–1810, 1999b

Ursano RJ, Fullerton CS, Epstein RS, et al: Acute and chronic posttraumatic stress disorder in motor vehicle accident victims. Am J Psychiatry 156:589–595, 1999a

van der Kolk BA: The compulsion to repeat the trauma: reenactment, revictimization, and masochism. Psychiatr Clin North Am 12:389–411, 1989

Weissman MM, Wickramaratne P, Adams PB, et al: The relationship between panic disorder and major depression: a new family study. Arch Gen Psychiatry 50:767–780, 1993

Wittchen HU, Carter RM, Pfister H, et al: Disabilities and quality of life in pure and comorbid generalized anxiety disorder and major depression in a national survey. Int Clin Psychopharmacol 15:319–328, 2000

Wittchen HU, Zhao S, Kessler RC, et al: DSM-III-R generalized anxiety disorder in the National Comorbidity Survey. Arch Gen Psychiatry 51:355–364, 1994

Woodruff R, Pitts FN Jr: Monozygotic twins with obsessional illness. Am J Psychiatry 20:1075–1080, 1964

Yehuda R, Schmeidler J, Wainberg M, et al: Vulnerability to posttraumatic stress disorder in adult offspring of Holocaust survivors. Am J Psychiatry 155:1163–1171, 1998a

Yehuda R, McFarlane AC, Shalev AY: Predicting the development of posttraumatic stress disorder from the acute response to a traumatic event. Biol Psychiatry 44:1305–1313, 1998b

2

DIAGNOSIS AND DIFFERENTIAL DIAGNOSIS

■ DIAGNOSING THE ANXIETY DISORDERS

Panic Disorder

DSM-II (American Psychiatric Association 1968) described an ill-defined condition of *anxiety neurosis*—a term first coined by Freud in 1895 (Breuer and Freud 1893–1895/1955)—that included any patient with chronic tension, excessive worry, frequent headaches, or recurrent anxiety attacks. However, subsequent findings began to show that discrete spontaneous panic attacks might be qualitatively dissimilar to other chronic anxiety states. For example, over the years, patients with panic attacks were found to be unique in their panic-induction responsiveness to sodium lactate infusion, familial aggregation, development of agoraphobia, and treatment response to tricyclic antidepressants. Thus DSM-III (American Psychiatric Association 1980) and subsequent DSM-III-R (American Psychiatric Association 1987) divided the category of *anxiety neurosis* into *panic disorder* and *generalized anxiety disorder (GAD)*.

The DSM-IV-TR (American Psychiatric Association 2000) criteria for panic attack are presented in Table 2–1. In a panic

---

TABLE 2–1.   **DSM-IV-TR criteria for panic attack**

Note: A panic attack is not a codable disorder. Code the specific diagnosis in which the panic attack occurs (e.g., 300.21 panic disorder with agoraphobia).

A discrete period of intense fear or discomfort, in which four (or more) of the following symptoms developed abruptly and reached a peak within 10 minutes:

   (1) palpitations, pounding heart, or accelerated heart rate
   (2) sweating
   (3) trembling or shaking
   (4) sensations of shortness of breath or smothering
   (5) feeling of choking
   (6) chest pain or discomfort
   (7) nausea or abdominal distress
   (8) feeling dizzy, unsteady, lightheaded, or faint
   (9) derealization (feelings of unreality) or depersonalization (being
         detached from oneself)
   (10) fear of losing control or going crazy
   (11) fear of dying
   (12) paresthesias (numbness or tingling sensations)
   (13) chills or hot flushes

---

attack, a person experiences the sudden onset of overwhelming fear, terror, apprehension, and a sense of impending doom and typically thinks he or she is dying, having a heart attack, "going crazy," or losing control. Several of a group of associated symptoms, mostly physical, are also experienced: dyspnea, palpitations, chest pain or discomfort, sensations of choking or smothering, dizziness or feeling of unsteadiness, feelings of unreality (derealization and/or depersonalization), paresthesias, hot and cold flashes, sweating, faintness, and trembling or shaking. Attacks typically last from 5 to 20 minutes, but (rarely) an attack can last as long as an hour.

Panic disorder is subdivided in DSM-IV-TR, as in DSM-III-R, into 1) panic disorder with agoraphobia and 2) panic disorder without agoraphobia—depending on whether there is any secondary phobic avoidance (see Tables 2–2 and 2–3). DSM-IV (American

TABLE 2–2.	**DSM-IV-TR criteria for panic disorder with agoraphobia**

A. Both (1) and (2):

   (1) recurrent unexpected panic attacks

   (2) at least one of the attacks has been followed by 1 month (or more) of one (or more) of the following:

      (a) persistent concern about having additional attacks

      (b) worry about the implications of the attack or its consequences (e.g., losing control, having a heart attack, "going crazy")

      (c) a significant change in behavior related to the attacks

B. The presence of agoraphobia

C. The panic attacks are not due to the direct physiological effects of a substance (e.g., a drug of abuse, a medication) or a general medical condition (e.g., hyperthyroidism).

D. The panic attacks are not better accounted for by another mental disorder, such as social phobia (e.g., occurring on exposure to feared social situations), specific phobia (e.g., on exposure to a specific phobic situation), obsessive-compulsive disorder (e.g., on exposure to dirt in someone with an obsession about contamination), posttraumatic stress disorder (e.g., in response to stimuli associated with a severe stressor), or separation anxiety disorder (e.g., in response to being away from home or close relatives).

Psychiatric Association 1994) clarified several issues regarding the diagnosis and differential diagnosis of panic disorder that had remained obscure in the DSM-III-R. For example, it is well known that panic attacks occur not only in panic disorder but in other anxiety disorders as well (e.g., specific phobia, social phobia, and posttraumatic stress disorder [PTSD]). In these other disorders, panic attacks are situationally bound or cued—that is, they occur exclusively in the context of the feared situation. DSM-IV clarified the confusion by explicitly presenting the criteria for panic attack (Table 2–1) independently of panic disorder (Tables 2–2 and 2–3) and specifying that a panic attack can be unexpected (uncued), situationally bound (cued), or situationally predisposed.

TABLE 2–3.	**DSM-IV-TR criteria for panic disorder without agoraphobia**

A. Both (1) and (2):

    (1) recurrent unexpected panic attacks

    (2) at least one of the attacks has been followed by 1 month (or more) of one (or more) of the following:

        (a) persistent concern about having additional attacks

        (b) worry about the implications of the attack or its consequences (e.g., losing control, having a heart attack, "going crazy")

        (c) a significant change in behavior related to the attacks

B. Absence of agoraphobia

C. The panic attacks are not due to the direct physiological effects of a substance (e.g., a drug of abuse, a medication) or a general medical condition (e.g., hyperthyroidism).

D. The panic attacks are not better accounted for by another mental disorder, such as social phobia (e.g., occurring on exposure to feared social situations), specific phobia (e.g., on exposure to a specific phobic situation), obsessive-compulsive disorder (e.g., on exposure to dirt in someone with an obsession about contamination), posttraumatic stress disorder (e.g., in response to stimuli associated with a severe stressor), or separation anxiety disorder (e.g., in response to being away from home or close relatives).

Using DSM-IV-TR, the diagnosis of panic disorder is made when a patient experiences recurrent panic attacks that are discrete and unexpected and that are followed by a month of persistent anticipatory anxiety or behavioral change. Although many persons experience occasional, or a few, panic attacks in their lifetime, the diagnosis of panic disorder is made only when the attacks occur with some regularity and frequency, although, genetically, panic disorder and any lifetime history of panic attacks may be related (Torgensen 1983). Finally, these attacks are not secondary to a known organic factor or due to another mental disorder. The differential diagnosis from other anxiety disorders that present with panic attacks can sometimes be complicated. Clinical judgment regarding the preponderant clinical pattern is called for in making the differential diagnosis in such cases. For example, if panic attacks occur almost exclusively in social contexts, the diagnosis of social phobia may be warranted. If they are clearly cued by social contexts, but also extensively occur in other situations or uncued, both diagnoses—panic disorder and social phobia—may be appropriate.

In typical onset of panic disorder, persons are engaged in some ordinary aspect of life when suddenly their heart begins to pound and they cannot catch their breath. They feel dizzy, light-headed, and faint and are convinced they are about to die. Panic disorder patients are usually young adults, most likely in their third decade, but they can be much younger or older. Not uncommonly, the first panic attack occurs in the context of a life-threatening illness or accident, in the loss of a close interpersonal relationship, or during separation from family. Patients who are developing hyperthyroidism can experience the first flurry of attacks at this time. Attacks can also begin in the immediate postpartum period. Finally, many patients have reported experiencing their first attacks while taking drugs of abuse—especially marijuana, lysergic acid diethylamide (LSD), cocaine, and amphetamines. However, even when these concomitant conditions are resolved, the attacks often continue unabated, suggesting that psychological or physical stressors may act as triggers to provoke the beginning of panic in people who are already predisposed. Often, the first panic attack is terrifying, and it is not unusual for persons experiencing a first attack to rush to the nearest emergency department, where routine laboratory tests, electrocardiography, and physical examination are performed. Typically, the findings of the medical workup are negative, patients are told that there is nothing physically wrong, and (it is hoped) they are informed that they experienced a panic attack.

Some patients do not progress in their illness beyond the point of continuing to have unexpected panic attacks. However, most patients develop some degree of anticipatory anxiety and phobic avoidance as a consequence of the experience of repetitive panic attacks. The patient comes to dread experiencing an attack and—in the intervals between attacks—starts worrying about doing so. This situation can progress until the level of fearfulness and autonomic hyperactivity in the interval between panic attacks almost approximates the level during the actual attack itself. Agoraphobia also frequently develops in response to panic attacks, leading to the DSM-IV-TR diagnosis of panic disorder with agoraphobia. The clinical picture in agoraphobia consists of multiple and varied fears and avoidance behaviors that center on three main themes: fear of leaving home, fear of being alone, and fear of being away from home in situations in which one can feel trapped, embarrassed, or helpless. Typical agoraphobic fears include the use of public transportation (buses, trains, subways, airplanes); being in crowds, theaters, elevators, restaurants, supermarkets, department stores; waiting in line; or traveling a distance from home. In agoraphobia at its worst, patients may be completely housebound, fearful of leaving home without a companion or even of staying home alone. The effect of a trusted companion on phobic behavior is a very interesting aspect of agoraphobia. Some patients who are unable to leave the house alone can travel long distances and partake of many activities if accompanied by a spouse, family member, or close friend.

Generalized Anxiety Disorder

As mentioned above, DSM-III first delineated generalized anxiety disorder (GAD), pulling it out of the broader preexistent category of anxiety neurosis of DSM-II. Currently, GAD is the main diagnostic category for prominent and chronic anxiety in the absence of panic disorder. The essential feature of this syndrome, according to DSM-IV-TR, is persistent anxiety lasting at least 6 months. The symptoms of this type of anxiety fall within two broad categories: 1) apprehensive expectation and worry and 2) physical symptoms. Patients with GAD are constantly worried over trivial matters, fearful, and anticipating the worst. Muscle tension, restlessness, feeling "keyed up," difficulty in concentrating, insomnia, irritability, and fatigue are typical signs of GAD. (These signs became the symptom criteria for GAD in DSM-IV, after a number of studies identified the physical symptoms that are the most distinctive and characteristic of GAD.) It turns out that motor tension and hypervigilance better differentiate GAD from other anxiety states than does autonomic hyperactivity (Marten et al. 1993; Starcevic et al. 1994). The DSM-IV-TR criteria for GAD simplify the cumbersome somatic symptom list previously found in DSM-III-R. In addition, DSM-IV-TR specifies that the diagnosis of GAD is excluded when anxiety or worrying occur exclusively in relation to other major Axis I disorders. We now know that clinicians must be cautious and conservative in applying this criterion, because, as described in Chapter 1, "Epidemiology," there are now compelling data demonstrating that even in the presence of high comorbidity of GAD with other anxiety and mood disorders, GAD is clearly a discrete disorder in terms of its onset, course, and associated impairment. Finally, DSM-IV-TR sharpens the distinction between GAD and everyday anxiety by specifying that in GAD the worry must be clearly excessive, pervasive, difficult to control, and associated with marked distress or impairment. In summary, then, the diagnosis of GAD is made when a patient experiences at least 6 months of chronic anxiety and excessive worry (although typically the patient's history presents a much more chronic pattern). At least three of six physical symptoms must also be present. Finally, the chronic anxiety must not be secondary to another Axis I disorder or a specific organic factor. The DSM-IV-TR criteria for GAD are presented in Table 2–4.

Phobias

A phobia is defined as a persistent and irrational fear of a specific object, activity, or situation that results in a compelling desire to avoid the dreaded object, activity, or situation (i.e., *phobic stimulus*). The fear is recognized by the individual as excessive or unreasonable in proportion to the actual dangerousness of the object, activity, or situation. Irrational fears and avoidance behavior are seen in a number of psychiatric disorders. However, in DSM-IV-TR the diagnosis of phobic disorder is made only when single or multiple phobias are the predominant aspect of the clinical picture and a source of significant distress to the individual, and not the result of another mental disorder.

TABLE 2–4.   **DSM-IV-TR criteria for generalized anxiety disorder**

A.   Excessive anxiety and worry (apprehensive expectation), occurring more days than not for at least 6 months, about a number of events or activities (such as work or school performance).

B.   The person finds it difficult to control the worry.

C.   The anxiety and worry are associated with three (or more) of the following six symptoms (with at least some symptoms present for more days than not for the past 6 months).   **Note:** Only one item is required in children.

   (1)   restlessness or feeling keyed up or on edge
   (2)   being easily fatigued
   (3)   difficulty concentrating or mind going blank
   (4)   irritability
   (5)   muscle tension
   (6)   sleep disturbance (difficulty falling or staying asleep, or restless unsatisfying sleep)

D.   The focus of the anxiety and worry is not confined to features of an Axis I disorder, e.g., the anxiety or worry is not about having a panic attack (as in panic disorder), being embarrassed in public (as in social phobia), being contaminated (as in obsessive-compulsive disorder), being away from home or close relatives (as in separation anxiety disorder), gaining weight (as in anorexia nervosa), having multiple physical complaints (as in somatization disorder), or having a serious illness (as in hypochondriasis), and the anxiety and worry do not occur exclusively during posttraumatic stress disorder.

E.   The anxiety, worry, or physical symptoms cause clinically significant distress or impairment in social, occupational, or other important areas of functioning.

F.   The disturbance is not due to the direct physiological effects of a substance (e.g., a drug of abuse, a medication) or a general medical condition (e.g., hyperthyroidism) and does not occur exclusively during a mood disorder, a psychotic disorder, or a pervasive developmental disorder.

Phobias were classified in DSM-I (American Psychiatric Association 1952) under the rubric phobic reaction and in DSM-II as phobic neurosis. No subtypes were listed in either edition, reflecting the assumption of a qualitative unity implicit in the psychoanalytic model of phobias. DSM-III markedly differed from the previous editions in classifying distinct subtypes of phobias, suggesting a qualitative distinction between these subtypes. This distinction between agoraphobia, social phobia, and miscellaneous specific phobias (listed under the disorder name *simple phobia*) stemmed from empirical findings, including behavioral treatment studies by Marks (1969) and pharmacological treatment studies by Klein (1964). These three major categories of phobias were maintained in DSM-III-R and later in DSM-IV and DSM-IV-TR. In DSM-III-R, agoraphobia was subdivided into panic disorder with agoraphobia and agoraphobia without history of panic disorder, emphasizing the primacy of panic when the two conditions coexist. This classification was maintained in DSM-IV and in DSM-IV-TR.

The major changes in the phobic disorders instituted in DSM-IV (and maintained in DSM-IV-TR), in relation to DSM-III-R, were as follows. In agoraphobia without history of panic disorder, it was specified that the condition centers on the fear of developing incapacitating symptoms, typically in characteristic situations. It was also specified that agoraphobia related to embarrassment over a medical illness is a diagnosis that can be made subject to clinical judgment. The two major changes in social phobia and in specific phobia were similar for the two disorders. First, it was made explicit that panic attacks can occur as a feature of these phobias and that therefore clinical judgment is needed in order to make the differential diagnosis between panic disorder with agoraphobia and social or specific phobia. Second, specific phobia was divided into types, because new evidence had accumulated demonstrating that phenomenology, natural history, and treatment response may differ according to type. The generalized type of social phobia was retained as in DSM-III-R. The DSM-IV-TR diagnostic criteria for agoraphobia without history of panic disorder, social phobia, and specific phobia are presented in Tables 2–5, 2–6, and 2–7, respectively.

TABLE 2–5.	DSM-IV-TR criteria for agoraphobia without history of panic disorder

A. The presence of agoraphobia related to fear of developing panic-like symptoms (e.g., dizziness or diarrhea).

B. Criteria have never been met for panic disorder.

C. The disturbance is not due to the direct physiological effects of a substance (e.g., a drug of abuse, a medication) or a general medical condition.

D. If an associated general medical condition is present, the fear described in Criterion A is clearly in excess of that usually associated with the condition.

Social Phobia

In social phobia, the patients' central fear is that they will act in such a way as to humiliate or embarrass themselves in front of others. Persons with social phobia fear and often avoid a variety of situations in which they would be required to interact with others or to perform a task in front of other people. Typical social phobias are of speaking, eating, or writing in public; using public lavatories; and attending social gatherings or interviews. In addition, a common fear on the part of people with social phobia is that other people will detect and ridicule their anxiety in social situations. An individual may have one, limited, or numerous social fears, and is therefore classified in one of three subtypes: fear of public speaking, fear of other circumscribed social situations, or generalized. Social phobia is described as generalized if the social fear encompasses most social situations, and this subtype is an overall more serious and impairing condition. Generalized social phobia can be reliably diagnosed as a subtype. Compared with nongeneralized social phobia, generalized social phobia has an earlier age at onset, patients are more often single and have more interactional fears, and it has a greater comorbidity with atypical depression and alcoholism (Mannuzza et al. 1995).

As in specific phobia, the anxiety in social phobia is stimulus-bound. When forced or surprised into the phobic situation, the indi-

TABLE 2–6.   **DSM-IV-TR criteria for social phobia**

A. A marked and persistent fear of one or more social or performance situations in which the person is exposed to unfamiliar people or to possible scrutiny by others. The individual fears that he or she will act in a way (or show anxiety symptoms) that will be humiliating or embarrassing.   **Note:** In children, there must be evidence of the capacity for age-appropriate social relationships with familiar people and the anxiety must occur in peer settings, not just in interactions with adults.

B. Exposure to the feared social situation almost invariably provokes anxiety, which may take the form of a situationally bound or situationally predisposed panic attack.   **Note:** In children, the anxiety may be expressed by crying, tantrums, freezing, or shrinking from social situations with unfamiliar people.

C. The person recognizes that the fear is excessive or unreasonable.   **Note:** In children, this feature may be absent.

D. The feared social or performance situations are avoided or else are endured with intense anxiety or distress.

E. The avoidance, anxious anticipation, or distress in the feared social or performance situation(s) interferes significantly with the person's normal routine, occupational (academic) functioning, or social activities or relationships, or there is marked distress about having the phobia.

F. In individuals under age 18 years, the duration is at least 6 months.

G. The fear or avoidance is not due to the direct physiological effects of a substance (e.g., a drug of abuse, a medication) or a general medical condition and is not better accounted for by another mental disorder (e.g., panic disorder with or without agoraphobia, separation anxiety disorder, body dysmorphic disorder, a pervasive developmental disorder, or Schizoid Personality disorder).

H. If a general medical condition or another mental disorder is present, the fear in Criterion A is unrelated to it, e.g., the fear is not of stuttering, trembling in Parkinson's disease, or exhibiting abnormal eating behavior in anorexia nervosa or bulimia nervosa.

Specify if:

   Generalized: if the fears include most social situations (also consider the additional diagnosis of avoidant personality disorder)

TABLE 2–7. **DSM-IV-TR criteria for specific phobia**

A. Marked and persistent fear that is excessive or unreasonable, cued by the presence or anticipation of a specific object or situation (e.g., flying, heights, animals, receiving an injection, seeing blood).

B. Exposure to the phobic stimulus almost invariably provokes an immediate anxiety response, which may take the form of a situationally bound or situationally predisposed panic attack. **Note:** In children, the anxiety may be expressed by crying, tantrums, freezing, or clinging.

C. The person recognizes that the fear is excessive or unreasonable. **Note:** In children, this feature may be absent.

D. The phobic situation(s) is avoided or else is endured with intense anxiety or distress.

E. The avoidance, anxious anticipation, or distress in the feared situation(s) interferes significantly with the person's normal routine, occupational (or academic) functioning, or social activities or relationships, or there is marked distress about having the phobia.

F. In individuals under age 18 years, the duration is at least 6 months.

G. The anxiety, panic attacks, or phobic avoidance associated with the specific object or situation are not better accounted for by another mental disorder, such as obsessive-compulsive disorder (e.g., fear of dirt in someone with an obsession about contamination), posttraumatic stress disorder (e.g., avoidance of stimuli associated with a severe stressor), separation anxiety disorder (e.g., avoidance of school), Social phobia (e.g., avoidance of social situations because of fear of embarrassment), panic disorder with agoraphobia, or agoraphobia without history of panic disorder.

Specify type:

Animal Type
Natural Environment Type (e.g., heights, storms, water)
Blood-Injection-Injury Type
Situational Type (e.g., airplanes, elevators, enclosed places)
Other Type (e.g., fear of choking, vomiting, or contracting an illness; in children, fear of loud sounds or costumed characters)

vidual experiences profound anxiety accompanied by a variety of somatic symptoms. Interestingly, different anxiety disorders tend to be characterized by their own constellation of most-prominent somatic symptoms. For example, palpitations and chest pain or pressure are more common in panic attacks, whereas sweating, blushing, and dry mouth are more common in social anxiety (Amies et al. 1983; Reich et al. 1988). Actual panic attacks may also occur in persons with social phobia in response to feared social situations. Blushing is the cardinal physical symptom characteristic of social phobia, whereas commonly encountered cognitive constellations include tendencies toward self-focused attention, negative self-evaluation regarding social performance, difficulty gauging non-verbal aspects of one's behavior, discounting of social competence in positive interactions, and a positive bias toward appraising others' social performance (Alden and Wallace 1995).

Persons who have only limited social fears may be functioning well overall and may be relatively asymptomatic unless confronted with the necessity of entering their phobic situation. When faced with this necessity, they are often subject to intense anticipatory anxiety. Multiple social fears, on the other hand, can lead to chronic demoralization, social isolation, and disabling vocational and interpersonal impairment. Often, alcohol and sedative drugs are used to alleviate at least the anticipatory component of this anxiety disorder, and in some persons this practice can lead to abuse. In a study that systematically compared people who had public-speaking phobia with people who had generalized social phobia, those with generalized social phobia were found to be younger; to be less educated; and to have greater rates of anxiety, depression, fears of negative social evaluation, and unemployment (Heimberg et al. 1990).

Specific Phobia

Specific phobia is circumscribed fear of specific objects, situations, or activities. The syndrome has three components: 1) an anticipatory anxiety that is brought on by the possibility of confrontation with the phobic stimulus, 2) the central fear itself, and 3) the avoidance behavior by which the individual minimizes anxiety. In specific phobia, the fear is usually not of the object, situation, or activity itself, but of some dire outcome that the individual believes may result from contact with that object, situation, or activity. For example, persons with snake phobia are afraid that they will be bitten; those who have claustrophobia, that they will suffocate or be trapped in an enclosed space; those with driving phobia are afraid of accidents. These fears are excessive, unreasonable, and enduring, so that although most persons with specific phobia will readily acknowledge that they know there is really nothing to be afraid of, reassuring them of this knowledge does not diminish their fear.

In DSM-IV, for the first time, subtypes of specific phobia were adopted: natural environment (e.g., storms); animal (e.g., insects); blood-injection-injury; situational (e.g., being in cars, in elevators, on bridges); and other (e.g., choking, vomiting). The validity of such distinctions is supported by data showing that these subtypes tend to differ with respect to age at onset, mode of onset, familial aggregation, and physiological responses to the phobic stimulus (Curtis and Thyer 1983; Fyer et al. 1990; Himle et al. 1991; Ost 1987). A comparable structure was found in child and adolescent specific phobia, clustering into three subtypes (Muris et al. 1999).

Obsessive-Compulsive Disorder

The essential features of obsessive-compulsive disorder (OCD) are obsessions and/or compulsions. The criteria for OCD in DSM-IV-TR are presented in Table 2–8. The terminology of *obsessions* or *compulsions* is sometimes used more broadly to characterize conditions that are not true OCD. Although some activities—such as eating, sexual activity, gambling, or drinking—when engaged in excessively may be referred to as "compulsive," these activities are distinguished from true compulsions in that they are typically experienced as pleasurable and ego-syntonic, at least in the moment (although their consequences may become increasingly unpleasant and ego-dystonic over time). Obsessive brooding, ruminations, or

---

TABLE 2–8. **DSM-IV-TR criteria for obsessive-compulsive disorder**

A. Either obsessions or compulsions:

Obsessions as defined by (1), (2), (3), and (4):

(1) recurrent and persistent thoughts, impulses, or images that are experienced, at some time during the disturbance, as intrusive and inappropriate and that cause marked anxiety or distress

(2) the thoughts, impulses, or images are not simply excessive worries about real-life problems

(3) the person attempts to ignore or suppress such thoughts, impulses, or images, or to neutralize them with some other thought or action

(4) the person recognizes that the obsessional thoughts, impulses, or images are a product of his or her own mind (not imposed from without as in thought insertion)

Compulsions as defined by (1) and (2):

(1) repetitive behaviors (e.g., hand washing, ordering, checking) or mental acts (e.g., praying, counting, repeating words silently) that the person feels driven to perform in response to an obsession, or according to rules that must be applied rigidly

(2) the behaviors or mental acts are aimed at preventing or reducing distress or preventing some dreaded event or situation; however, these behaviors or mental acts either are not connected in a realistic way with what they are designed to neutralize or prevent or are clearly excessive

B. At some point during the course of the disorder, the person has recognized that the obsessions or compulsions are excessive or unreasonable. **Note:** This does not apply to children.

C. The obsessions or compulsions cause marked distress, are time consuming (take more than 1 hour a day), or significantly interfere with the person's normal routine, occupational (or academic) functioning, or usual social activities or relationships.

TABLE 2–8.   **DSM-IV-TR criteria for obsessive-compulsive disorder** *(continued)*

D. If another Axis I disorder is present, the content of the obsessions or compulsions is not restricted to it (e.g., preoccupation with food in the presence of an eating disorder; hair pulling in the presence of trichotillomania; concern with appearance in the presence of body dysmorphic disorder; preoccupation with drugs in the presence of a substance use disorder; preoccupation with having a serious illness in the presence of hypochondriasis; preoccupation with sexual urges or fantasies in the presence of a paraphilia; or guilty ruminations in the presence of major depressive disorder).

E. The disturbance is not due to the direct physiological effects of a substance (e.g., a drug of abuse, a medication) or a general medical condition.

Specify if:

With Poor Insight: if, for most of the time during the current episode, the person does not recognize that the obsessions and compulsions are excessive or unreasonable

---

preoccupations, typically characteristic of depression, can be very unpleasant but are distinguished from true obsessions because they are not as senseless or intrusive and the individual regards them as meaningful although often excessive and biased toward self-blame and self-denigration.

Obsessive and compulsive symptoms have been recognized for centuries and were first described in the psychiatric literature by Esquirol in 1838 (Rachman and Hodgson 1980). Obsessional thoughts were defined by Karl Westphal in 1878 as ideas that occur in an otherwise intact intelligence, are not caused by an affective state, are against the will of the person, and come into the foreground of consciousness (Westphal 1878).

There are several presentations of OCD based on symptom clusters. One group includes patients with obsessions about dirt and contamination, whose rituals center on compulsive washing and avoidance of contaminated objects. A second group includes patients with pathological counting and compulsive checking. A third group includes purely obsessional patients with no compulsions. Primary obsessional slowness is evident in another group, in whom slowness is the predominant symptom; patients may spend many hours every day getting washed, dressed, and eating breakfast, and life goes on at an extremely slow speed. Some OCD patients, called hoarders, are unable to throw anything out for fear they might someday need something they discarded.

In DSM-IV-TR, OCD is classified among the anxiety disorders because 1) anxiety is often associated with obsessions and resistance to compulsions, 2) anxiety or tension is often immediately relieved by yielding to compulsions, and 3) OCD often occurs in association with other anxiety disorders. However, compulsions decrease anxiety only transiently, and the nature of the fears in OCD is distinct from those of other anxiety disorders. Certain diagnostic disputes regarding OCD were investigated in the DSM-IV field trial and led to some clarifications and changes in the criteria. Even though obsessions are typically experienced as ego-dystonic, there is a wide range of insight in patients with OCD. Although most patients have some degree of insight, about 5% are convinced that their obsessions and compulsions are reasonable (Foa et al. 1995). On the basis of this finding, DSM-IV specified a poor-insight type if, for most of the time during the current episode, the person does not recognize that the obsessions and compulsions are excessive or unreasonable. DSM-IV also made explicit that compulsions can be either behavioral or mental. Mental rituals are encountered in the great majority of OCD patients and, like behavioral compulsions, are intended to reduce anxiety or prevent harm. Although more than 90% of patients with OCD have features of both obsessions and compulsions, about 20%–30% are bothered mainly by obsessions, 20% by compulsions, and 50% by both (Akhtar et al. 1975; Foa et al. 1995; Rachman and Hodgson 1980; Welner et al. 1976).

OCD usually begins in adolescence or early adulthood but can begin prior to that time; 31% of first episodes occur by ages 10–15 years, with 75% developing by age 30 (Black 1974). In most cases, no particular stress or event precipitates the onset of OCD symptoms, and an insidious onset is followed by a chronic and often progressive course. However, some patients describe a sudden onset of symptoms. This sudden onset of symptoms is particularly true of patients with a neurological basis for their illness. There is evidence of OCD associated with the 1920s encephalitis epidemic (Meyer-Gross and Steiner 1921), abnormal birth events (for OCD in the child) (Capstick and Seldrup 1977), onset following head injury (McKeon et al. 1984) and seizures (Kehl and Marks 1986), and, more recently, streptococcal infections (Leonard and Swedo 2001). There are also reports of new onset of OCD during pregnancy (Neziroglu et al. 1992).

An obsession is an intrusive, unwanted mental event, usually evoking anxiety or discomfort. Obsessions can be thoughts, ideas, images, sounds, ruminations, convictions, fears, or impulses, and they often have an aggressive, sexual, religious, disgusting, or nonsensical content. Obsessional ideas are repetitive thoughts that interrupt the regular train of thought, whereas obsessional images are often vivid visual experiences. Much obsessive thinking involves horrific ideas, such as of committing blasphemy, rape, murder, or child molestation. Obsessional convictions are often characterized by an element of magical thinking, such as "Step on the crack, break your mother's back." Obsessional ruminations may involve prolonged, excessive, and inconclusive thinking about metaphysical questions. Obsessional fears often involve dirt or contamination; they differ from phobias because they are present in the absence of the phobic stimulus, exaggerate the likely presence of the phobic stimulus, and can be irrational in the methods applied to counteract the fear. Other common obsessional fears involve harm coming to oneself or to others as a consequence of one's misdoing—such as one's home catching on fire because the stove was not checked, or running over a pedestrian because of careless driving. Patients resist and control their obsessions in varying degrees, and significant impairment in functioning can result. *Resistance* is the struggle against an impulse or intrusive thought, whereas *control* is the patient's actual success in diverting the thinking process.

Another hallmark of obsessive thinking involves lack of certainty or persistent doubting. In contrast to patients with mania or psychosis, who manifest premature certainty, OCD patients are unable to achieve a reasonable sense of certainty about the accuracy of incoming sensory information. Are my hands clean? Is the door locked? Is the fertilizer poisoning the water supply? Compulsive rituals such as excessive washing or checking appear to arise from this excessive lack of certainty, and consist of a misguided attempt to increase certainty.

A compulsive ritual is a behavior that usually reduces discomfort but is carried out in a pressured or rigid fashion. Such behavior may include rituals involving washing, checking, repeating, avoiding, striving for completeness, and being meticulous. Washers represent about 25%–50% of most OCD samples (Akhtar et al. 1975; Rachman and Hodgson 1980; Rasmussen and Tsuang 1986). These persons are concerned with dirt, contaminants, or germs and may spend many hours a day washing their hands or showering. They may also attempt to avoid contaminating themselves with feces, urine, or vaginal secretions. Checkers have pathological doubt and thus compulsively check to see if they have, for example, run over someone with their car, left the door unlocked, or left the stove on. Checking often fails to resolve the doubt and in some cases may actually exacerbate it. In the DSM-IV field trial, washing and checking were the two most common groups of compulsions.

Although slowness results from most rituals, it is the major feature of the rare and disabling syndrome of primary obsessional slowness. It may take several hours for the obsessionally slow individual to get dressed or get out of the house. This slowness may be a response to a lack of certainty as well. These persons may have little anxiety despite their obsessions and rituals.

Mental compulsions are also quite common and should be inquired about directly, because they could go undetected if the clinician asks only about behavioral rituals. Such patients, for example, may replay over and over in their minds past conversations with others to make sure they did not somehow incriminate themselves.

Similarly, they may replay over and over in their minds recent actions to ensure, for example, that they did not make mistakes. In the DSM-IV OCD field trials, 80% of patients with OCD had both behavioral and mental compulsions, and mental compulsions were the third most common type after checking and washing.

Although all these distinct OCD symptom clusters exist, symptoms can overlap or develop sequentially over time. One study examined the distribution and grouping of obsessive-compulsive symptoms in about 300 OCD patients and found that a total of four symptom dimensions accounted for more than 60% of variance: 1) obsessions and checking, 2) symmetry and ordering, 3) cleanliness and washing, and 4) hoarding (Leckman et al. 2001). Such subtypes may prove useful in the research of possible genetic, neurobiological, or treatment-response heterogeneity within the disorder.

Posttraumatic Stress Disorder

PTSD was first introduced in DSM-III, spurred in part by the increasing recognition of posttraumatic conditions in veterans of the Vietnam War. The current DSM-IV-TR criteria for PTSD are presented in Table 2–9. As in DSM-III-R, the disorder continues to be classified with the anxiety disorders, and the major criteria—an extreme precipitating stressor, intrusive symptoms, avoidance, and hyperarousal—have been maintained. (The DSM-III-R descriptor of the traumatic event as one "outside the range of usual human experience" was deemed vague and unreliable and was eliminated.) New duration criteria were also established, subdividing the disorder into acute and chronic.

Not all investigators agree that PTSD belongs with the anxiety disorders. Although anxiety is a prominent symptom, so are depression and dissociation. The necessity of a precipitating stressor or trauma in diagnosing the disorder differs from other anxiety disorders and is more reminiscent of reactive or trauma-spectrum conditions, such as brief reactive psychosis, pathological bereavement, and adjustment disorders. *International Classification of Diseases*, 10th Revision (ICD-10; World Health Organization 1992), for

TABLE 2–9.   **DSM-IV-TR criteria for posttraumatic stress disorder**

A.   The person has been exposed to a traumatic event in which both of the following were present:

   (1)   the person experienced, witnessed, or was confronted with an event or events that involved actual or threatened death or serious injury, or a threat to the physical integrity of self or others.

   (2)   the person's response involved intense fear, helplessness, or horror.   **Note:** In children, this may be expressed instead by disorganized or agitated behavior.

B.   The traumatic event is persistently reexperienced in one (or more) of the following ways:

   (1)   recurrent and intrusive distressing recollections of the event, including images, thoughts, or perceptions.   **Note:** In young children, repetitive play may occur in which themes or aspects of the trauma are expressed.

   (2)   recurrent distressing dreams of the event.   **Note:** In children, there may be frightening dreams without recognizable content.

   (3)   acting or feeling as if the traumatic event were recurring (includes a sense of reliving the experience, illusions, hallucinations, and dissociative flashback episodes, including those that occur on awakening or when intoxicated).   **Note:** In young children, trauma-specific reenactment may occur.

   (4)   intense psychological distress at exposure to internal or external cues that symbolize or resemble an aspect of the traumatic event

   (5)   physiological reactivity on exposure to internal or external cues that symbolize or resemble an aspect of the traumatic event

C.   Persistent avoidance of stimuli associated with the trauma and numbing of general responsiveness (not present before the trauma), as indicated by three (or more) of the following:

   (1)   efforts to avoid thoughts, feelings, or conversations associated with the trauma

   (2)   efforts to avoid activities, places, or people that arouse recollections of the trauma

   (3)   inability to recall an important aspect of the trauma

   (4)   markedly diminished interest or participation in significant activities

TABLE 2–9.	**DSM-IV-TR criteria for posttraumatic stress disorder *(continued)***

    (5) feeling of detachment or estrangement from others

    (6) restricted range of affect (e.g., unable to have loving feelings)

    (7) sense of a foreshortened future (e.g., does not expect to have a career, marriage, children, or a normal life span)

D. Persistent symptoms of increased arousal (not present before the trauma), as indicated by two (or more) of the following:

    (1) difficulty falling or staying asleep

    (2) irritability or outbursts of anger

    (3) difficulty concentrating

    (4) hypervigilance

    (5) exaggerated startle response

E. Duration of the disturbance (symptoms in Criteria B, C, and D) is more than 1 month.

F. The disturbance causes clinically significant distress or impairment in social, occupational, or other important areas of functioning.

Specify if:

    Acute: if duration of symptoms is less than 3 months
    Chronic: if duration of symptoms is 3 months or more

Specify if:

    With Delayed Onset: if onset of symptoms is at least 6 months after the stressor

example, classifies all such disorders as stress-related. In acknowledgment of the spectrum of disorders stemming from severe stress, DSM-IV added acute stress disorder (ASD) to the anxiety disorders. ASD is similar to PTSD in the precipitating traumatic event and in symptomatology but is time-limited (lasting up to 1 month after the event). In addition, dissociative symptoms figure prominently in the definition of ASD, whereas they are not addressed in the PTSD description. It has now been well established by a number of studies, including prospective ones, that ASD is a highly reliable predictor of developing PTSD down the road; it may well be that the two disorders should not be defined as discrete disorders. In a study of persons who received mild traumatic brain injury in motor vehicle accidents, 82% of those who met ASD criteria were given the diagnosis of PTSD 6 months later (Bryant and Harvey 1998), as opposed to only 11% of those without ASD, and a steady 80% were still diagnosed with PTSD 2 years after the accident (Harvey and Bryant 2000).

Beyond the symptoms of PTSD as such, increasing attention has been drawn to an enduring constellation of traits that frequently develop in persons subjected to chronic and complex trauma, often as children but also possibly in adulthood. Investigators such as Herman and van der Kolk originally suggested that a discrete entity of complicated posttraumatic syndromes be recognized and designated as DESNOS (disorders of extreme stress not otherwise specified). This entity was characterized by a more complex clinical picture than "pure" PTSD, with lasting changes in identity, interpersonal relationships, and the sense of life's meaning (Herman and van der Kolk 1987; van der Kolk and Saporta 1991). Similar personality changes are recognized by ICD-10 and classified as "enduring personality change after catastrophic experience." Increasing attention has been drawn in the last decade to the concept of "trauma-spectrum" disorders—which can include admixtures of posttraumatic stress and dissociative, somatoform, and conversion symptoms—and the preferred classification approach to trauma-related conditions remains a subject of ongoing debate.

A soldier participates in the torture and murder of civilians. A passenger is the sole survivor of the crash of a commercial airliner. A woman is raped and severely beaten by an unknown assailant. The characteristic symptoms that can develop following such traumatic events center on reexperiencing of the trauma, avoidance and numbing, and increased autonomic arousal. The trauma is reexperienced in recurrent painful, intrusive recollections, flashbacks, nightmares, or intense emotional and physiologic reactions to reminders of the trauma. Psychic numbing or emotional anesthesia is manifest by diminished investment in the external world, with feelings of being detached from other people, loss of interest in usual activities, and inability to feel positive emotions such as intimacy, tenderness, or sexual interest. Persons and situations reminiscent of the original trauma may be systematically avoided. Dissociative states may occur, lasting from minutes to days, in which the individual is in a dreamlike, unreal state with hazy memory and a distorted sense of time. Symptoms of excessive autonomic arousal may include irritability and anger, an exaggerated startle response, difficulty concentrating, hypervigilance, and insomnia. In addition to the three major symptom criteria, other PTSD symptoms include guilt about having survived, guilt about not having prevented the traumatic experience, depression, anxiety, panic attacks, shame, helplessness, and rage. There may be prolonged episodes of intense and poorly modulated affect, resulting in explosive, hostile outbursts or impulsive behaviors. Other accompanying or complicating symptoms associated with PTSD may include substance abuse, self-injurious behaviors, suicide attempts, occupational impairment, and interference with interpersonal relationships.

■ DIFFERENTIAL DIAGNOSIS

Panic Disorder

The differential diagnosis of panic disorder is summarized in Table 2–10. Psychiatric conditions that involve pathological anxiety can at times make the differential diagnosis of panic disorder difficult. Sometimes the differentiation of primary anxiety disorder from depression can be problematic. Patients with major depression often manifest signs of anxiety and might even have frank panic attacks that occur only during bouts of depression. Conversely, patients with panic disorder, if untreated for significant amounts of time, routinely become demoralized as the impact of the illness progressively restricts their ability to pursue their usual lives, and this state may be reminiscent of depression. However, panic disorder can become complicated by secondary major depression, or vice versa. An overall elevated comorbidity between panic disorder and depression further complicates the picture.

TABLE 2–10. **Differential diagnosis of panic disorder**

Anxious depression
Somatization disorder with paniclike physical complaints
Social phobia with socially cued panic attacks
GAD with severe symptoms or during peak periods
PTSD with intense physiologic response to reminders of the trauma
Agoraphobia secondary to conditions other than panic disorder
  (depression, PTSD, paranoia, psychosis)
Obsessional tension states of near-panic severity
Depersonalization disorder
Personality disorder with anxiety symptoms
Hyperthyroidism
Hypothyroidism
Mitral valve prolapse
Pheochromocytoma
Vestibular disorders
Panic attack associated with substance use or withdrawal (cocaine use,
  alcohol withdrawal)

Note. GAD = generalized anxiety disorder; PTSD = posttraumatic stress disorder.

Although the differentiation of anxiety from depression can at times strain even the most experienced clinician, several points are helpful. Patients with panic disorder generally do not demonstrate the full range of vegetative symptoms that are seen in depression. Thus, patients with anxiety usually have trouble falling asleep—rather than problems with early morning awakening—and do not lose their appetite. Diurnal mood fluctuation is uncommon in anxiety disorder. Perhaps of greatest importance is the fact that most patients with anxiety do not lose the capacity to enjoy things or to be cheered up as endogenously depressed patients do. The distinction between atypical depression and anxiety disorders is even more difficult because of the lack of typical endogenous features in atypical depression. However, although patients with atypical depression can also be cheered up, they tend to slump faster than patients with anxiety disorder.

The order of developing symptoms also differentiates depression from anxiety. In cases of panic disorder, anxiety symptoms usually precede any seriously altered mood. Patients can generally recall having anxiety attacks first, then becoming gradually more demoralized and "down." In depression, patients usually experience dysphoria first, with anxiety symptoms coming later.

Therefore, the clinician's task is to elicit the presenting symptoms of panic disorder and of depression, along with the patient's lifetime histories of the disorders and their temporal relationships to each other, to determine whether only one condition or both are present. If both, did one disorder serve as trigger to the other, or do the two disorders appear independent of each other?

A few other psychiatric conditions need to be differentiated from panic disorder. Patients with somatization disorder complain of a variety of physical ailments and discomforts, none of which are substantiated by physical or laboratory findings. Unlike panic disorder patients, patients with somatization disorder present with physical problems that do not usually occur in episodic attacks of multiple symptoms but are virtually constant and involve more limited symptoms.

Patients with depersonalization disorder have episodes of derealization and depersonalization without the other symptoms of a panic attack, and the dissociative symptoms tend to be recurrent or persistent, typically of much longer duration than that of a panic attack. However, panic attacks not infrequently involve depersonalization and derealization as prominent symptoms, and limited-symptom panic attacks in which only depersonalization and derealization are elicited as spontaneous symptoms before further probing could be confused with depersonalization disorder.

Although patients with panic disorder often fear they will "lose their minds" or "go crazy," psychotic illness is not an outcome of anxiety disorder. Reassuring the patient on this point is often the first step in a successful treatment, because patients who are not knowledgeable in this regard may truly fear that they will "go insane." It is important, however, not to overlook the possible presence of comorbid panic disorder in patients with psychotic disorders. Panic disorder could be missed either because patients with psychotic disorders are less likely to give clear accounts of their attacks or because these patients' reports of anxiety symptoms could be misattributed to psychotic anxiety surrounding paranoid or delusional fears.

Undoubtedly, some patients with anxiety disorders abuse alcohol and drugs such as sedatives in attempts at self-medication. Quitkin and Babkin (1982) found that after successful detoxification, a group of alcoholic patients with a prior history of panic disorder were treated with medication to block spontaneous panic attacks. These patients did not resume alcohol consumption once their panic attacks were eliminated.

With regard to the agoraphobic component of the disorder, widespread fears and avoidance of being along or of leaving home can also be seen in paranoid and psychotic states, posttraumatic stress disorder, and major depressive disorders. Psychotic states can be differentiated from agoraphobia by the presence of delusions, hallucinations, and thought process disorder. Although patients with agoraphobia might be afraid they are "going crazy," they do not exhibit psychotic symptomatology. Patients with PTSD typically have a clear history of trauma and may be avoiding various situations that are reminders of that trauma. Patients with depression can usually make the distinction that they are avoiding leaving their home not because they are fearful of symptoms that could occur if they go out, but because they have no motivation, interest, or energy to face their life or do things.

Sometimes individuals describe atypical panic attacks, the differential diagnosis of which need to be further explored. Patients who claim they have attacks that last a whole day may experience one of four patterns: 1) Some patients continue to feel anxious, agitated, and fatigued for several hours after the main portion of the attack has subsided. 2) At times, attacks occur, subside, and occur again in a wavelike manner. 3) The patient with so-called "long" panic attacks is often experiencing some other form of pathological anxiety, such as severe generalized anxiety, agitated depression, or obsessional tension of near-panic intensity. 4) In some cases, such severe anticipatory anxiety may develop over time in expectation of future panic attacks that the two—the anticipation and the actual attack—may blend together in a patient's description and be difficult to distinguish.

The patient may have a medical condition that should be considered in the differential diagnosis of panic disorder. Patients with either hyperthyroidism or hypothyroidism can present with anxiety unaccompanied by other signs or symptoms. For this reason, it is imperative that all patients complaining of anxiety undergo routine thyroid function tests, including an evaluation of the level of thyroid-stimulating hormone. It should be remembered, however, that thyroid disease can act as one of the predisposing triggers to panic disorder, so that even when thyroid disease is corrected, panic attacks might continue until specifically treated.

The relationship of mitral valve prolapse to panic disorder has attracted a great deal of attention over the years. This usually benign condition was shown by a number of investigators to occur more frequently in patients with panic disorder than in psychiatrically healthy subjects. However, screening of patients known to have mitral valve prolapse reveals no greater frequency of panic disorder than is found in the overall population. Although patients with mitral valve prolapse occasionally complain of palpitations, chest pain, light-headedness, and fatigue, the symptoms of a full-blown panic attack are rare. Panic disorder patients with mitral valve prolapse and those without the condition are similar in several important ways. Effectiveness or ineffectiveness of the treatment for panic attacks is not affected by the presence of a prolapsed valve. Patients with both mitral valve prolapse and panic disorder are just as sensitive to sodium lactate as are those with panic disorder alone. Some researchers have speculated that mitral valve prolapse and panic disorder may represent manifestations of the same underlying disorder of autonomic nervous system function (Gorman et al. 1981). Others have suggested that panic disorder, by creating intermittent states of high circulating catecholamine levels and tachycardia, actually causes mitral valve prolapse (Mattes 1981). There are reports that mitral valve prolapse might go away if the panic disorder is kept under control (Gorman et al. 1981). According to a meta-analysis of 21 studies, there does appear to be an association between panic disorder and mitral valve prolapse, although the possibility of publication bias favoring positive reports cannot be ruled out (Katerndahl 1993). In any event, it is clear that the presence of mitral valve prolapse in patients with panic disorder has little clinical or prognostic importance in the management of spontaneous panic attacks. What the presence of mitral valve prolapse may tell us about the underlying etiology of panic disorder is a question currently under vigorous investigation.

Hyperparathyroidism occasionally manifests as anxiety symptoms, warranting laboratory tests of serum calcium level before definitive diagnosis is made. A variety of cardiac conditions can initially appear as anxiety symptoms, although in most cases the patient with a cardiac condition complains prominently of chest pain, skipped beats, or palpitations. Ischemic heart disease and arrhythmias—especially paroxysmal atrial tachycardia—should be ruled out by electrocardiography. Pheochromocytoma is a rare, usually benign tumor of the adrenal medulla that secretes catecholamines in episodic bursts. During an active phase, the patient characteristically experiences flushing, tremulousness, and anxiety. Blood pressure is usually elevated during the active phase of catecholamine secretion but not at other times. Therefore, merely finding blood pressure in a normal range does not rule out a pheochromocytoma. If this condition is suspected, the diagnosis is made by collection of urine for 24 hours and determining the catecholamine metabolite concentration. In a study of patients with confirmed pheochromocytoma, about half met the criteria for the physical symptoms of panic attacks, but none had panic disorder, because they did not experience terror during the attacks and did not develop anticipatory anxiety or agoraphobia; these distinctions are very helpful in making the differential diagnosis (Starkman et al. 1990).

Disease of the vestibular nerve can cause episodic bouts of vertigo, light-headedness, nausea, and anxiety that mimic panic attacks. Rather than merely feeling dizzy, such patients often experience true vertigo in which the room seems to spin in one direction during each attack. Otolaryngology consultation is warranted when this condition is suspected. Some patients with panic disorder complain primarily of dizziness or unsteadiness. Whether they make up a distinct subgroup of panic disorder patients with definite neurotologic abnormalities is currently under study.

Although many patients believe their anxiety disorder is caused by reactive hypoglycemia, there is no scientific proof at present that hypoglycemia is ever a cause of any psychiatric disturbance. Glucose tolerance tests are not helpful in establishing hypoglycemia as the cause of anxiety, because up to 40% of the general population will have a random low blood glucose level during a routine glucose tolerance test. The only convincing way to establish hypoglycemia as a cause of anxiety symptoms would be to document a low blood glucose level at the same time the patient is symptomatic, and this has not been done.

Generalized Anxiety Disorder

The differential diagnosis of GAD is summarized in Table 2–11. As previously mentioned, patients with GAD may at times have peaks in the severity of their anxiety that reach panic-like proportions, sometimes in the context of vulnerable situations triggered in the context of an underlying personality disorder. GAD can be differentiated from panic disorder by the absence of frank, clear-cut panic attacks. In addition, the fatigue, motor tension, and vigilance characteristic of GAD are different from the prominent autonomic symptoms of panic. OCD patients may also experience chronic anxiety that may be reminiscent of GAD, but this anxiety typically revolves around their obsessional fears rather than exaggerated worries of everyday life. Patients with social phobia who exist in socially demanding settings and do not have much avoidance may find themselves, consequently, in a frequent state of anxiety that may be reminiscent of GAD. However, cognitive elaboration of the content of the anxiety usually helps make the differential diagnosis. Additionally, the physical manifestations of social phobia center more on palpitations, blushing, and tremor. Finally, the symptoms

TABLE 2–11.	**Differential diagnosis of generalized anxiety disorder**

Anxious depression
Panic attacks or anticipatory anxiety
Social phobia
PTSD-related hyperarousal symptoms
Obsessional fearfulness
Hypochondriasis
Paranoid anxiety associated with psychosis or personality disorder

Note. PTSD = posttraumatic stress disorder.

of GAD, such as motor tension, apprehensive expectation, vigilance, and scanning, are also present in PTSD. However, the onset and course of the illnesses differ: GAD has an insidious or gradual onset and a course that fluctuates with environmental stressors, whereas PTSD has an acute onset after usually clear trauma, often followed by a chronic course. Phobic avoidant symptoms, which are absent in GAD, are often present in PTSD.

Social Phobia

Before the diagnosis of phobic disorder can be made, the presence of other disorders that may cause irrational fears and avoidance behaviors must be ruled out. The differential diagnosis of social phobia is summarized in Table 2–12.

Avoidance of social situations is seen as part of avoidant, schizoid, and paranoid personality disorders; agoraphobia; OCD; depressive disorders; schizophrenia; and paranoid disorders. Persons with paranoid disorders fear that something unpleasant will be done to them by others and that others have malignant intent. In contrast, persons with social phobia fear that they themselves will act inappropriately and cause their own embarrassment or humiliation. In avoidant personality disorder, the central fear is also rejection, ridicule, or humiliation by others. The distinction between this entity and generalized social phobia may be conceptual or semantic, and its validity remains a subject of dispute. When patients who

---

TABLE 2–12. **Differential diagnosis of social phobia**

Personality disorder, such as avoidant, schizoid, paranoid

Axis I paranoid disorder, such as paranoid schizophrenia or paranoid delusional disorder

Depression-related social withdrawal secondary to anhedonia or feelings of defectiveness

OCD-related fears exacerbated in social settings (e.g., contamination)

Panic disorder with phobic avoidance not limited to social situations

Deficits or impaired social skills associated with schizophrenia and related disorders

Body dysmorphic disorder with secondary social phobia

Note.   OCD = obsessive-compulsive disorder.

---

avoid social situations are automatically labeled as having avoidant personalities, the clinician may be led away from potentially useful pharmacotherapy and behavioral treatment. Patients with social phobia have difficulties with social settings, whereas patients with avoidant personality tend to have difficulty establishing close individual relationships regardless of social context.

Some patients with agoraphobia say that they are afraid they will embarrass themselves by losing control if they panic while in a social situation. Unlike patients with social phobia, patients with agoraphobia experience panic attacks that also occur in situations not involving scrutiny or evaluation by others. If panic attacks occur only in social situations and the agoraphobia is limited to social settings, social phobia is the more appropriate diagnosis.

Interpersonal anxiety or fears of humiliation leading to social avoidance are not diagnosed as social phobia when they occur in the context of schizophrenia, schizophreniform or brief reactive psychoses, and major depressive disorder. Patients with psychotic vulnerabilities and massive social isolation or poor interpersonal skills may occasionally be mistaken as having social phobia if they are seen when they are in nonpsychotic or prepsychotic phases of illness. Social withdrawal seen in depressive disorders is usually associated with a lack of interest or pleasure in the company of others, and depressive persons will have difficulty sustaining their usual mode of interaction rather than having a fear of scrutiny. In contrast, persons with social phobia generally express the wish to be able to interact appropriately with others and anticipate pleasure in this eventuality.

Obsessive-Compulsive Disorder

The diagnosis of OCD is usually clear-cut, but occasionally it can be more difficult to distinguish OCD from depression, psychosis, phobias, or severe obsessive-compulsive personality disorder. All other Axis I disorders can be comorbid with OCD; however, for the diagnosis of OCD to be made, the OCD symptoms must not be merely secondary to another disorder (e.g., thoughts about food in the presence of an eating disorder, or guilty thoughts in the presence of major depression).

In some cases the course of OCD may more closely resemble that of schizophrenia, with chronic debilitation, decline, and profound impairment in social and occupational functioning. Sometimes it is difficult to distinguish between an obsession (i.e., contamination) and a delusion (i.e., being poisoned). Typically, an obsession is ego-dystonic, resisted, and recognized by the patient as having an internal origin. A delusion is not resisted and is believed to be external. OCD patients, however, may lack insight, and obsessions in 12% of cases may become delusions (Gittleson 1966). Yet longitudinal studies show that OCD patients are not at increased risk of developing schizophrenia (Black 1974). DSM-IV-TR allows the diagnosis of both disorders simultaneously. In fact, up to 25% of patients with schizophrenia might have features of OCD. Thus the presence of significant obsessive-compulsive symptoms in a schizophrenic patient should not be neglected and warrants separate treatment.

Frequently, patients with OCD have complicating depressions, and these patients may be difficult to distinguish from depressed patients who have complicating obsessive symptoms. Patients with psychotic depression, agitated depression, or premorbid obsessional features prior to depression are particularly likely to develop prominent obsessional thinking when depressed (Gittleson 1966). These "secondary" obsessions often involve aggressive, guilty, self-denigrating mood-congruent themes, but the distinction between primary and secondary obsessions rests on the order of occurrence. In addition, depressive ruminations—in contrast to pure obsessions—are often focused on a past incident rather than a current or future event and are rarely resisted or counteracted by compulsive rituals.

A close connection exists between OCD and phobic disorders. OCD patients who are compulsive cleaners appear very similar to persons with phobia, and are mislabeled "germ phobics" by some. Both have avoidant behavior, both show intense subjective and autonomic response to focal stimuli, and both are said to respond to similar behavioral interventions (Rachman and Hodgson 1980). Both have excessive fear, although disgust is prominent in OCD patients and not in patients with phobia. However, OCD patients can never entirely avoid obsession, always imagine unlikely scenarios, and have irrational concepts of how to neutralize their fears, whereas patients with phobia have more focal, external, and realistic stimuli, which they can then successfully avoid.

Patients with OCD who experience high levels of anxiety may describe paniclike episodes, but these episodes are secondary to obsessions and do not arise spontaneously. In contrast to patients with anxiety disorder, OCD patients do not experience anxiety attacks when lactate infusions are administered (Gorman et al. 1985). The differential diagnosis of OCD is summarized in Table 2–13.

Posttraumatic Stress Disorder

The diagnosis of PTSD is usually not difficult if there is a clear history of exposure to a traumatic event, followed by symptoms of intense anxiety lasting at least 1 month, with arousal and stimulation of the autonomic nervous system, numbing of responsiveness, and avoidance or reexperiencing of the traumatic event. However, a wide variety of anxiety, depressive, somatic, and behavioral symptoms for which the relationship between their onset and the trau-

TABLE 2–13. **Differential diagnosis of obsessive-compulsive disorder**

Eating disorder with obsessions surrounding food and weight

Body dysmorphic disorder with obsessions about body appearance other than weight

Hypochondriasis with obsessions related to feared illnesses

Panic disorder or generalized anxiety disorder (if obsessional anxiety is severe)

Obsessive ruminations of depressions (typically mood-congruent)

Severe obsessive-compulsive personality disorder

Paranoid psychosis (e.g., delusions of poisoning rather than fears of contamination)

Social phobia (if social situations are avoided because they exacerbate OCD)

Impulse control disorders (repetitive behaviors associated with pleasure or gratification (e.g., compulsive gambling, compulsive spending, or compulsive sexual behavior)

Note. OCD = obsessive-compulsive disorder.

matic event is less clear-cut may easily lead to misdiagnosis. It is always crucial when establishing the PTSD diagnosis to clearly assess the onset of symptoms as subsequent to the trauma. In addition, a high rate of comorbidity can often lead to the additional diagnosis of panic, depression, or GAD along with the PTSD, because it is well established that the preexistence of such conditions renders individuals at higher risk of developing PTSD after a trauma, followed by a recurrence or intensification of their preexisting mood and anxiety disorders.

In particular, there is much overlap between PTSD and major mood disorders. Symptoms such as psychic numbing, irritability, sleep disturbance, fatigue, anhedonia, impairments in family and social relationships, anger, concern with physical health, and pessimistic outlook may occur in both disorders. In some veteran outreach populations, 70%–80% of patients meet the diagnostic criteria for both disorders. Major depression is a frequent complication of PTSD; when it occurs, it must be treated aggressively, because comorbidity carries an increased risk of suicide. If major depression develops secondary to PTSD, both disorders should be diagnosed. Dysthymic symptoms are frequently secondary to PTSD, but if symptoms are sufficiently severe, the additional diagnosis of dysthymic disorder should be made.

Following a traumatic event, patients may be aversively conditioned to the surroundings of the trauma and develop a phobia of objects, surroundings, or situations that remind them of the trauma itself. Patients with phobia experience anxiety in the feared situation, whereas avoidance is accompanied by anxiety reduction that reinforces the avoidant behavior. In PTSD, the phobia may be symptomatically similar to specific phobia, but the nature of the trigger as a specific reminder of the trauma, and the symptom cluster of PTSD, distinguish this condition from specific phobia.

Patients with PTSD may also experience panic attacks. In some patients, panic attacks predate the PTSD, or do not occur exclusively in the context of stimuli reminiscent of the traumatic event. In some patients, however, panic attacks develop after the PTSD and are cued solely by traumatic stimuli. If the panic attacks are extensive and meet the criteria for the disorder, the diagnosis should be made.

Adjustment disorders are maladaptive reactions to identifiable psychosocial pressures. Signs and symptoms may include a wide variety of disturbances and emerge within 3 months of the stressful event. If symptoms are of sufficient severity to meet other Axis I criteria, then the diagnosis of adjustment disorder is not made. Adjustment disorder can be diagnosed in the presence of another Axis I or Axis II disorder if one of those disorders does not account for the symptoms that occur as a result of the stressful event. Adjustment disorder differs from PTSD, because the stressor is usually less severe and within the range of common experience, and the characteristic symptoms of PTSD—such as reexperiencing the trauma—are absent. The prognosis of full recovery in adjustment disorder is usually excellent.

Compensation neurosis, factitious disorder, and malingering involve conscious deception and feigning of illness, although the motivation for each condition differs. Patients with factitious disorder may present with physical or psychological symptoms; the feigning of symptoms is under voluntary control; and the motivation is to assume the "patient" role. Chronic factitious disorder with physical symptoms (e.g., Munchausen syndrome) involves frequent visits to the physician, recurrent hospitalizations, and may involve surgical interventions. PTSD differs from factitious disorder by its absence of fabricated symptoms, its acute onset following a trauma, and the absence of a bizarre pretraumatic medical and psychiatric history.

Malingering involves the conscious fabrication of an illness for the purpose of achieving a definite goal such as money, compensation, and so forth. Malingerers often reveal an inconsistent history, unexpected symptom clusters, a history of antisocial behavior and substance abuse, and a chaotic lifestyle, and there is often a discrepancy between history, claimed distress, and objective data.

Following acute physical traumas, head trauma, or concussion, organic mental disorder must be ruled out when diagnosing PTSD, because such events have important treatment implications. Mild concussions may leave no immediate, apparent neurological signs but may have residual long-term effects on mood and concentration. A careful evaluation of the nature of any head trauma—including medical records and witnesses' observations, evaluation of mental status, neurological examination, and (if indicated) laboratory tests—is essential in a diagnostic workup. Malnutrition, which may occur during prolonged stressful periods, can lead to organic brain syndromes. Survivors of death camps can have symptoms of an organic mental disorder—failing memory, difficulty concentrating, emotional lability, headaches, and vertigo. Other causes of organic mental disorder may occasionally mimic PTSD if anxiety, depression, personality changes, or abnormal behaviors are present. Aberrant thoughts, memories, senses, or level of consciousness, or focal neurological signs, would suggest an organic mental disorder.

Organic mental disorders that could mimic PTSD include organic personality syndrome, delirium, amnestic syndrome, organic hallucinosis, or organic intoxication and withdrawal states. In addition, patients with PTSD may cope by excessive use of alcohol, drugs, caffeine, or tobacco, and thus present with a combination of organic and psychological factors—in which case each concomitant disorder should be diagnosed. The differential diagnosis of PTSD is summarized in Table 2–14.

TABLE 2–14. **Differential diagnosis of posttraumatic stress disorder**

Depression after trauma (numbing and avoidance may be present, but not hyperarousal or intrusive symptoms)

Panic disorder (if panic attacks are not limited to reminders or triggers of the trauma)

GAD (may have symptoms similar to PTSD hyperarousal)

Agoraphobia (if avoidance is not directly trauma-related)

Specific phobia (if avoidance is not directly trauma-related)

Adjustment disorder (usually has less severe stressor and different symptoms)

ASD (if less than 1 month has elapsed since trauma)

Dissociative disorders (if prominent dissociative symptoms are present)

Factitious disorders or malingering (especially if secondary gain is apparent)

Note. ASD = acute stress disorder; GAD = generalized anxiety disorder; PTSD = posttraumatic stress disorder.

■ REFERENCES

Akhtar S, Wig NN, Varma VK, et al: A phenomenological analysis of symptoms in obsessive-compulsive neurosis. Br J Psychiatry 127:342–348, 1975

Alden LE, Wallace ST: Social phobia and social appraisal in successful and unsuccessful social interactions. Behav Res Ther 33:497–505, 1995

American Psychiatric Association: Diagnostic and Statistical Manual: Mental Disorders. Washington, DC, American Psychiatric Association, 1952

American Psychiatric Association: Diagnostic and Statistical Manual of Mental Disorders, 2nd Edition. Washington, DC, American Psychiatric Association, 1968

American Psychiatric Association: Diagnostic and Statistical Manual of Mental Disorders, 3rd Edition. Washington, DC, American Psychiatric Association, 1980

American Psychiatric Association: Diagnostic and Statistical Manual of Mental Disorders, 3rd Edition, Revised. Washington, DC, American Psychiatric Association, 1987

American Psychiatric Association: Diagnostic and Statistical Manual of Mental Disorders, 4th Edition. Washington, DC, American Psychiatric Association, 1994

American Psychiatric Association: Diagnostic and Statistical Manual of Mental Disorders, 4th Edition, Text Revision. Washington, DC, American Psychiatric Association, 2000

Amies PL, Gelder MG, Shaw PM: Social phobia: a comparative clinical study. Br J Psychiatry 142:174–179, 1983

Black A: The natural history of obsessional neurosis, in Obsessional States. Edited by Beech HK. London, Methuen Press, 1974, pp 19–54

Breuer T, Freud S: Studies on hysteria (1893–1895), in The Standard Edition of the Complete Psychological Works of Sigmund Freud, Vol 2. Edited by Strachey J. London, Hogarth Press, 1955, pp 1–319

Bryant RA, Harvey AG: Relationship between acute stress disorder and posttraumatic stress disorder following mild traumatic brain injury. Am J Psychiatry 155:625–629, 1998

Capstick N, Seldrup V: Obsessional states: a study in the relationship between abnormalities occurring at birth and subsequent development of obsessional symptoms. Acta Psychiatr Scand 56:427–439, 1977

Curtis GC, Thyer B: Fainting on exposure to phobic stimuli. Am J Psychiatry 140:771–774, 1983

Foa EB, Kozak MJ, Goodman WK, et al: DSM-IV field trial: obsessive-compulsive disorder. Am J Psychiatry 152:90–96, 1995

Fyer AJ, Mannuzza S, Gallops MS, et al: Familial transmission of simple phobias and fears: a preliminary report. Arch Gen Psychiatry 47:252–256, 1990

Gittleson NL: The effect of obsessions on depressive psychosis. Br J Psychiatry 112:253–259, 1966

Gorman JM, Fyer AF, Gliklich J, et al: Effect of imipramine on prolapsed mitral valves of patients with panic disorder. Am J Psychiatry 138:977–978, 1981

Gorman JM, Liebowitz MR, Fyer AJ, et al: Lactate infusions in obsessive-compulsive disorder. Am J Psychiatry 142:864–866, 1985

Harvey AG, Bryant RA: Two-year prospective evaluation of the relationship between acute stress disorder and posttraumatic stress disorder following mild traumatic brain injury. Am J Psychiatry 157:626–628, 2000

Heimberg RG, Hope DA, Dodge CS, et al: DSM-III-R subtypes of social phobia: comparison of generalized social phobics and public speaking phobics. J Nerv Ment Dis 178:172–179, 1990

Herman JL, van der Kolk BA: Traumatic antecedents of borderline personality disorder, in Psychological Trauma. Edited by van der Kolk BA. Washington, DC, American Psychiatric Press, 1987, pp 111–126

Himle JA, Crystal D, Curtis GC, et al: Mode of onset of simple phobia subtypes: further evidence of heterogeneity. Psychiatry Res 36:37–43, 1991

Katerndahl DA: Panic and prolapse. Meta-analysis. J Nerv Ment Dis 181:539–544, 1993

Kehl PA, Marks IM: Neurological factors in obsessive-compulsive disorder: two case reports and a review of the literature. Br J Psychiatry 149:315–319, 1986

Klein DF: Delineation of two drug responsive anxiety syndromes. Psychopharmacologia 5:397–408, 1964

Leckman JF, Zhang H, Alsobrook JP, et al: Symptom dimensions in obsessive-compulsive disorder: toward quantitative phenotypes. Am J Med Genet 105(1):28–30, 2001

Leonard HL, Swedo SE: Paediatric autoimmune neuropsychiatric disorders associated with streptococcal infection (PANDAS). Int J Neuropsychopharmacol 4(2):191–198, 2001

Mannuzza S, Schneier FR, Chapman TF, et al: Generalized social phobia. Reliability and validity. Arch Gen Psychiatry 52:230–237, 1995

Marks IM: Fears and Phobias. New York, Academic Press, 1969

Marten PA, Brown TA, Barlow DH, et al: Evaluation of the ratings comprising the associated symptom criterion of DSM-III-R generalized anxiety disorder. J Nerv Ment Dis 181:676–682, 1993

Mattes J: More on panic disorder and mitral valve prolapse (letter). Am J Psychiatry 138:1130, 1981

McKeon J, McGuffin P, Robinson P: Obsessive-compulsive neurosis following head injury: a report of four cases. Br J Psychiatry 144:190–192, 1984

Meyer-Gross W, Steiner G: Zentralblatt fur die Gesamte Neurologie und Psychiatrie 73:287–289, 1921

Muris P, Schmidt H, Meckelbach H: The structure of specific phobia symptoms among children and adolescents. Behav Res Ther 37:863–868, 1999

Neziroglu F, Anemone R, Yaryura-Tobias JA: Onset of obsessive-compulsive disorder in pregnancy. Am J Psychiatry 149:947–950, 1992

Ost LG: Age of onset of different phobias. J Abnorm Psychol 96:223–229, 1987

Quitkin F, Babkin J: Hidden psychiatric diagnosis in the alcoholic, in Alcoholism and Clinical Psychiatry. Edited by Soloman J. New York, Plenum, 1982, pp 129–140

Rachman SJ, Hodgson RJ: Obsessions and Compulsions. Englewood Cliffs, NJ, Prentice-Hall, 1980

Rasmussen SA, Tsuang MT: Clinical characteristics and family history in DSM-III obsessive compulsive disorder. Am J Psychiatry 143:317–322, 1986

Reich J, Noyes R, Yates W: Anxiety symptoms distinguishing social phobia from panic and generalized anxiety disorders. J Nerv Ment Dis 176:510–513, 1988

Skre I, Onstad S, Torgensen S, et al: A twin study of DSM-III-R anxiety disorders. Acta Psychiatr Scand 88:85–92, 1993

Starcevic V, Fallon S, Uhlenhuth EH: The frequency and severity of generalized anxiety disorder symptoms. Toward a less cumbersome conceptualization. J Nerv Ment Dis 182:80–84, 1994

Torgensen S: Genetic factors in anxiety disorders. Arch Gen Psychiatry 40:1085–1089, 1983

Starkman MN, Cameron OG, Nesse RM, et al: Peripheral catecholamine levels and the symptoms of anxiety: studies in patients with and without pheochromocytoma. Psychosom Med 52:129–142, 1990

van der Kolk BA, Saporta J: The biological response to psychic trauma: mechanisms and treatment of intrusion and numbing. Anxiety Research 4:199–212, 1991

Welner A, Reich T, Robins E, et al: Obsessive-compulsive neurosis: record, family, and follow-up studies. Compr Psychiatry 17:527–539, 1976

Westphal K: Ueber Zwangsverstellungen [Obsessional thoughts]. Arch Psychiatr Neurol 8:734–750,1878

World Health Organization: International Classification of Diseases, 10th Revision. Geneva, World Health Organization, 1992

3

COURSE AND PROGNOSIS

■ PANIC DISORDER

The course of panic disorder without treatment is highly variable. At the present time there is no reliable way to know which patients will develop, for example, agoraphobia. Panic disorder seems to have a waxing and waning course in which spontaneous recovery occurs, only to be followed months to years later by a resurgence of attacks. At the extreme, some patients become completely housebound for decades. Treatment aimed at blocking the occurrence of the attacks is appropriate at any point in the course of the illness when such attacks are occurring. Results are frequently dramatic. Pharmacologic blockade of panic attacks early in the illness, before phobic avoidance has become an ingrained way of life, often leads to complete remission. Even years into the illness, effective control of the attacks can lead to resolution of anticipatory anxiety and phobias without other treatment. However, a substantial number of patients with major phobic avoidance remain anxious and frightened of confronting feared situations even after the attacks have been blocked, and these patients require other forms of intervention in addition.

A 7-year follow-up study examined prognostic factors in naturalistically treated patients with panic disorder. Although patients had generally good outcomes, there were several predictors of poorer outcome, including greater severity of panic attacks and agoraphobia, longer duration of illness, comorbid major depression, separation from a parent by death or divorce, high interpersonal sensitivity, low social class, and single marital status (Noyes et al. 1993). Another long-term outcome study, covering a 5-year period, had fairly optimistic findings—34% of patients were recovered, 46% were minimally impaired, and 20% remained moderately to severely impaired. The most notable predictor of poor outcome was an anxious-fearful personality type, and the second most notable was poor response to initial treatment (O'Rourke et al. 1996). Still another large outcome study showed that fewer than 20% of panic disorder patients remained seriously agoraphobic or disabled. Baseline frequency of panic attacks, initial pharmacologic treatment, and continuous use of medication were all unrelated to outcome, whereas longer duration of illness and more severe initial avoidance were predictors of unfavorable outcome (Katschnig et al. 1995). Course and prognosis of panic disorder are summarized in Table 3–1.

TABLE 3–1.	**Course and prognosis of panic disorder**
Course	Variable, typically with periods of exacerbations and remissions
Outcome	$1/3$ of patients fully recover
	$1/2$ of patients have minimal impairment
	$1/5$ of patients, or fewer, have moderate to severe impairment
Predictors of poor prognosis[a]	
	More severe panic attacks
	More severe agoraphobia
	Longer duration of illness
	Comorbid major depression
	History of separation from parent (death, divorce)
	Low social class
	Anxious personality type
	High degree of interpersonal sensitivity
	Poor response to initial treatment
	Single marital status

Note. Fractional figures for outcome are approximate.

[a] Data from Katschnig et al. 1995; Noyes et al. 1993; O'Rourke et al. 1996.

An earlier study showed a higher incidence of premature death, due to cardiovascular illness and suicide, among patients with panic disorder than among healthy subjects without psychiatric or medical problems (Coryell et al. 1982). However, each of the patients in the study had had psychiatric hospitalization at some point, raising a question as to whether they constituted a more severely ill group of patients than is generally encountered in clinical practice. The increased death rate from cardiovascular illness described in the clinical study by Coryell et al. was partly supported in an epidemiologic investigation by Weissman and her group (1990). In the Weissman study, patients with panic disorder had a substantially higher risk of strokes than patients with other psychiatric disorders (although several methodologic limitations to the study were identified). The one cardiovascular abnormality that was found in the Weissman study to occur at a higher rate in patients with panic disorder is mitral valve prolapse. This association could conceivably explain a higher incidence of cardiovascular-related death in patients with panic disorder; however, mitral valve prolapse itself is rarely a cause of premature death or major morbidity. One other possible explanation for increased cardiovascular and cerebrovascular risk in patients with panic disorder may be related to lifestyle. Patients with panic disorder tend to live relatively sedentary lives, some reporting that vigorous physical exercise precipitates their panic attacks, leading them to avoid exertion. Heavy cigarette smoking, alcoholism, and poor diets could also contribute to an increased risk in panic patients. Alternatively, left ventricular enlargement and increased risk of thromboembolic events were contemplated to account for the association between panic disorder and increased risk of cardiovascular and cerebrovascular complications (Weissman et al. 1990); however, this consideration remains speculative.

The putative association between panic disorder and increased suicide risk has received much attention in the last decade. Initially it was thought that the association might be due to the fact that patients with panic disorder are more prone than are people without psychiatric problems to major depressive disorder and to alcoholism at some point in their lives. However, Allgulander and Lavori (1991) conducted a large retrospective survey in Sweden and found an increased suicide risk in panic disorder in the absence of comorbid diagnoses. Epidemiologic data further supported this finding in the Epidemiologic Catchment Area (ECA) study in which the lifetime rate of suicide attempts by persons with uncomplicated panic disorder was 7%—about the same as the 7.9% rate by persons with uncomplicated major depression (Johnson et al. 1990). However, in a reanalysis of the ECA data, controlling for all comorbidity rather than one disorder at a time, an association between panic and suicide attempts could no longer be shown (Hornig and McNally 1995). In a clinical sample of panic disorder patients a 17% incidence of suicide attempts was found for those without comorbid major depression or substance abuse, but these patients did have other comorbidity with some depressive symptomatology and/or personality disorder (Lepine et al. 1993). The latest study of this issue (a 5-year prospective study) again concluded that there was no association between panic disorder and suicide risk in the absence of other risk factors (Warshaw et al. 2000). It does appear at this time that there is no direct link between uncomplicated panic disorder and suicide.

■ GENERALIZED ANXIETY DISORDER

In contrast to panic disorder, no overwhelming single event prompts the patient with generalized anxiety disorder (GAD) to seek help. Such patients seem only over time to develop the recognition that their experience of chronic tension, hyperactivity, worry, and anxiety is excessive. Often they will state that there has never been a time in their lives, as long as they can remember, when they were not anxious. GAD appears to be a more chronic condition than panic disorder, with fewer periods of spontaneous remission (Raskin et al. 1982; Woodman et al. 1999). Of GAD subjects followed over a 5-year period, only 18%–35% attained full remission (Woodman et al. 1999; Yonkers et al. 1996). Patients with GAD experience substantial interference with their lives, often seek professional help, and make substantial use of medications (Wittchen et al. 1994). GAD patients with an earlier onset of anxiety symptoms in the first two decades of life appear to be overall more impaired, to suffer from more severe anxiety that is not precipitated by specific stressful events, and to have histories of more childhood fears, disturbed family environments, and greater social maladjustment (Hoehn-Saric et al. 1993). As pointed out earlier, although GAD is commonly comorbid with major depression and other anxiety disorders, it still emerges as a clearly distinct entity (Brawman et al. 1993; Wittchen et al. 2000). Abuse of alcohol, barbiturates, and antianxiety medications is also common. Breslau and Davis (1985) showed that if GAD is persistent for 6 months, then the rate of comorbidity with depressive disorder is very high. Also, the probability of GAD remission over time is lower in the presence of comorbid depression (Yonkers et al. 1996). Contrary to panic disorder, which declines with old age, GAD appears to account for many of the anxiety states in late life, often comorbidly with medical illnesses (Flint 1994). In elderly patients with anxiety, it is particularly important to differentiate GAD from other anxiety states that could be related to delirium, dementia, psychosis, or depression or that could be manifestations of underlying medical illnesses.

■ SOCIAL PHOBIA

Social phobia has its onset mainly in adolescence and early adulthood, usually earlier than panic disorder with agoraphobia, and the course of the illness is typically highly chronic. Onset of symptoms is sometimes acute following a humiliating social experience, but much more often it is insidious over months or years and without a clear-cut precipitant. Frequently patients recall having had social phobia as teenagers, sometimes even in grade school. As shown by clinical studies, men are affected as often as women by social phobia—a difference from other anxiety disorders. This finding probably reflects who is more likely to seek treatment under societal role demands, because the prevalence rate of social phobia in the population at large shows it to be somewhat more common in women.

Social phobia is clearly a chronic and potentially highly impairing condition. More than half of social phobia patients report substantial impairment in some areas of their lives, independent of the degree of social support they have (Schneier et al. 1994; Stein and Kean 2000). Predictors of good outcome in social phobia include onset after age 11, absence of psychiatric comorbidity, and higher educational status (Davidson et al. 1993). In a recent, very large, retrospective survey of persons ages 15–64 years with lifetime social phobia, approximately half of the sample had recovered from their illness at the time of survey; data showed a median illness duration of 25 years. Important predictors of recovery were childhood social context (i.e., no siblings and small-town rearing), onset after age 7, minimal symptoms, and absence of comorbid health problems or depression, or health problems and depression that occurred before the onset of social phobia (DeWit et al. 1999). Course and prognosis of social phobia are summarized in Table 3–2.

TABLE 3–2.	**Course and prognosis of social phobia**
Course	Typically, early onset at or before adolescence and very chronic course
Outcome	About $\frac{1}{2}$ of patients found to be recovered after 25 years of illness
Predictors of poorer prognosis	Onset before ages 8–11 years Comorbid psychiatric disorder Lower educational status More symptoms at initial evaluation Comorbid health problems

■ SPECIFIC PHOBIA

In specific phobia, the typical age at onset varies according to the type of phobia. Animal phobias usually begin in childhood, whereas situational phobias tend to start later in life. Marks (1969) found a mean age at onset for animal phobias to be 4.4 years, whereas patients with situational phobias had a mean age at onset of 22.7 years.

Although systematic prospective studies are limited, it appears that specific phobias follow a chronic course unless treated. A recent study followed up specific phobia patients 10–16 years after an initial treatment and found that even among responders with complete initial recovery, about half were clinically symptomatic at follow-up. In addition, none of the patients who had not improved with the initial treatment were any better at the time of the follow-up. The study suggests that specific phobias might be resistant to treatment or often do not receive treatment (Lipsitz et al. 1999).

■ OBSESSIVE-COMPULSIVE DISORDER

Studies of the natural course of obsessive-compulsive disorder (OCD) suggest that in 24%–33% of patients the disorder has a fluctuating course, in 11%–14% it follows a phasic course with periods of complete remission, and in 54%–61% it has a constant or progressive course (Black 1974). Although prognosis for OCD has traditionally been considered to be poor, developments in behavioral and pharmacological treatments have considerably improved the prognosis. The disorder usually has a major impact on daily functioning, with some patients spending many waking hours consumed with their obsessions and rituals. Often, patients are socially isolated, marry at an older age, and have a high celibacy rate (particularly in males) and a low fertility rate. Compounding the situation, depression and anxiety are common complications of OCD.

Recently, a major follow-up study in Sweden followed the course of patients over a 40-year period, from approximately the 1950s to the 1990s, (Skoog and Skoog 1999). Findings were more optimistic than one might have expected, with improvement noted in 83% of patients. Of those, about half were fully or almost fully recovered. Importantly, predictors of worse outcome were earlier age at onset, a more chronic course at baseline, poorer social functioning at baseline, having both obsessions and compulsions, and magical thinking. In a recent study by the International Consortium of the Treatment of Refractory OCD, the patients who did not improve with treatment were those who had more severe illness, greater delusional severity, OCD with a more chronic course, and more comorbidity with bipolar and eating disorders (Hollander et al. 2002). In terms of acute treatment, the presence of hoarding obsessions and compulsions is associated with poorer response to medication treatment (Mataix-Cols et al. 1999). Course and prognosis of OCD are summarized in Table 3–3.

■ POSTTRAUMATIC STRESS DISORDER

Scrignar (1984) has divided the clinical course of posttraumatic stress disorder (PTSD) into three stages:

Stage I involves the response to trauma. Nonsusceptible persons can experience an adrenergic surge of symptoms immediately after the trauma but typically do not dwell on the incident. Predisposed persons have higher levels of anxiety and dissociation at initial evaluation, an exaggerated response to the trauma, and a preoccupation with the trauma.

TABLE 3–3.	Course and prognosis of obsessive-compulsive disorder
Course	Slightly more than $1/10$ of patients: phasic with periods of complete remission
	$1/4$ to $1/3$ of patients: fluctuating course
	$1/2$ of patients: constant or progressive illness
Outcome	Slightly more than $4/5$ of patients improve over 40 years
Predictors of worse prognosis	Early age at onset
	Longer duration of illness
	Presence of both obsessions and compulsions
	Poorer baseline social functioning
	Magical thinking and greater delusional severity
	Chronic course of illness
	Comorbid bipolar disorder or eating disorder

Note. Fractions are approximate.

If symptoms persist beyond 4–6 weeks, the patient enters *stage II*, or acute PTSD. Feelings of helplessness and loss of control, symptoms of increased autonomic arousal, "reliving" of the trauma, and somatic symptoms may occur. The patient's life becomes centered on the trauma, with subsequent changes in lifestyle, personality, and social functioning. Phobic avoidance, startle responses, and angry outbursts can occur.

In *stage III*, chronic PTSD develops, with disability, demoralization, and despondency. The patient's emphasis might change from preoccupation with the actual trauma to preoccupation with the physical disability resulting from the trauma. Somatic symptoms, chronic anxiety, and depression are common complications at this time, as well as substance abuse, disturbed family relations, and unemployment. Some patients might focus on compensation and lawsuits.

One study found that the full remission rate for chronic PTSD over a 5-year prospective period was only 18%, highlighting the frequent chronicity of the illness. History of alcohol abuse and childhood trauma was associated with a lower rate of remission (Zlotnick et al. 1999). Even when statistically correcting for comorbid psychiatric or medical disorders, researchers found that persons with PTSD manifest substantial impairment in major domains of living, such as physical limitations, unemployment, poor physical health, and diminished well-being. Thus, in patients with multiple disorders, it can be crucial to specifically target and treat PTSD if it is present (Zatzick et al. 1997).

Recent data show that the large majority of PTSD patients, more than 80%, have chronic PTSD (defined in DSM-IV-TR [American Psychiatric Association 2000] as PTSD having a duration of longer than 3 months); about 75% of patients with PTSD continue to be symptomatic at 6 months. Median time to remission of PTSD is about 2 years (Breslau et al. 1998). The National Comorbidity Survey revealed that the decline in PTSD symptoms is steeper over the first year, and more gradual subsequently (Kessler et al. 1995). Some persons, especially those exposed to assault or horrific events such as the Holocaust, can remain symptomatic for decades after the trauma. There are several factors predictive of greater chronicity (i.e., greater number of PTSD symptoms at initial evaluation, psychiatric history of other anxiety or mood disorders, greater numbing or hyperarousal in response to stressors, comorbid medical illnesses, and female sex) (Breslau and Davis 1992). Table 3–4 summarizes the course and prognosis of PTSD.

TABLE 3–4.	Course and prognosis of posttraumatic stress disorder
Course[a]	$^4/_5$ of patients: longer than 3 months
	$^3/_4$ of patients: longer than 6 months
	$^1/_2$ of patients: 2 years' duration
	Minority of patients: symptomatic for many years or for decades
Predictors of worse outcome	Greater number of PTSD symptoms
	Psychiatric history of other anxiety and mood disorders
	Higher degree of numbing or hyperarousal to stressors
	Comorbid medical illnesses
	Female sex
	Childhood trauma
	Alcohol abuse

Note. PTSD = posttraumatic stress disorder.
[a]Data from Breslau et al. 1998.

■ REFERENCES

Allgulander C, Lavori PW: Excess mortality among 3302 patients with "pure" anxiety neurosis. Arch Gen Psychiatry 48:599–602, 1991

American Psychiatric Association: Diagnostic and Statistical Manual of Mental Disorders, 4th Edition, Text Revision. Washington, DC, American Psychiatric Association, 2000

Black A: The natural history of obsessional neurosis, in Obsessional States. Edited by Beech HK. London, Methuen Press, 1974, pp 19–54

Brawman MO, Lydiard RB, Emmanuel N, et al: Psychiatric comorbidity in patients with generalized anxiety disorder. Am J Psychiatry 150:1216–1218, 1993

Breslau N, Davis GC: DSM-III generalized anxiety disorder: an empirical investigation of more stringent criteria. Psychiatry Res 15:231–238, 1985

Breslau N, Davis GC: Posttraumatic stress disorder in an urban population of young adults: risk factors for chronicity. Am J Psychiatry 149:671–675, 1992

Breslau N, Kessler RC, Chilcoat HD, et al: Trauma and posttraumatic stress disorder in the community: the 1996 Detroit Area Survey of Trauma. Arch Gen Psychiatry 55:626–632, 1998

Coryell W, Noyes R, Clancy J: Excess mortality in panic disorder: a comparison with primary unipolar depression. Arch Gen Psychiatry 39:701–703, 1982

Davidson JR, Hughes DL, George LK, et al: The epidemiology of social phobia: findings from the Duke Epidemiological Catchment Area Study. Psychol Med 23:709–718, 1993

DeWit DJ, Ogborne A, Offord DR, et al: Antecedents of the risk of recovery from DSM-III-R social phobia. Psychol Med 29:569–582, 1999

Flint AJ: Epidemiology and comorbidity of anxiety disorders in the elderly. Am J Psychiatry 151:640–649, 1994

Hoehn-Saric R, Hazlett RL, McLeod DR: Generalized anxiety disorder with early and late onset of anxiety symptoms. Compr Psychiatry 34:291–298, 1993

Hollander E, Bienstock C, Pallanti S, et al: Refractory obsessive-compulsive disorder: state-of-the-art treatment. J Clin Psychiatry 63 (suppl 6):20–29, 2002

Hornig CD, McNally RJ: Panic disorder and suicide attempt: a reanalysis of data from the Epidemiologic Catchment Area study. Br J Psychiatry 167:76–79, 1995

Johnson J, Weissman MM, Klerman GL: Panic disorder, comorbidity, and suicide attempts. Arch Gen Psychiatry 47:805–808, 1990

Katschnig H, Amering M, Stolk JM, et al: Long-term follow-up after a drug trial for panic disorder. Br J Psychiatry 167:487–494, 1995

Kessler RC, Sonnega A, Bromet E, et al: Posttraumatic stress disorder in the National Comorbidity Survey. Arch Gen Psychiatry 52:1048–1060, 1995

Lepine JP, Chignon JM, Teherani M: Suicide attempts in patients with panic disorder. Arch Gen Psychiatry 50:144–149, 1993

Lipsitz JD, Markowitz JC, Cherry S, et al: Open trial of interpersonal psychotherapy for the treatment of social phobia. Am J Psychiatry 156:1814–1816, 1999

Marks IM: Fears and Phobias. New York, Academic Press, 1969

Mataix-Cols D, Rauch SL, Manzo PA, et al: Use of factor-analyzed symptom dimensions to predict outcome with serotonin reuptake inhibitors and placebo in the treatment of obsessive-compulsive disorder. Am J Psychiatry 156:1409–1416, 1999

Noyes R Jr, Clancy J, Woodman C, et al: Environmental factors related to the outcome of panic disorder. A seven-year follow-up study. J Nerv Ment Dis 181:529–538, 1993

O'Rourke D, Fahy TJ, Brophy J, et al: The Galway study of panic disorder. III. Outcome at 5 to 6 years. Br J Psychiatry 168:462–469, 1996

Raskin M, Peeke HVS, Dickman W, et al: Panic and generalized anxiety disorders: developmental antecedents and precipitants. Arch Gen Psychiatry 39:687–689, 1982

Schneier FR, Heckelman LR, Garfinkel R, et al: Functional impairment in social phobia. J Clin Psychiatry 55:322–331, 1994

Scrignar CB: Post-Traumatic Stress Disorder: Diagnosis, Treatment, and Legal Issues. New York, Praeger, 1984

Skoog G, Skoog I: A 40-year follow-up of patients with obsessive-compulsive disorder. Arch Gen Psychiatry 56:121–127, 1999

Stein MB, Kean YM: Disability and quality of life in social phobia: epidemiologic findings. Am J Psychiatry 157:1606–1613, 2000

Warshaw MG, Dolan RT, Keller MB: Suicidal behavior in patients with current or past panic disorder: five years of prospective data from the Harvard/Brown Anxiety Research Program. Am J Psychiatry 157:1876–1878, 2000

Weissman MM, Markowitz JS, Ouellette R, et al: Panic disorder and cardiovascular/cerebrovascular problems: results from a community survey. Am J Psychiatry 147:1504–1508, 1990

Wittchen HU, Zhao S, Kessler RC, et al: DSM-III-R generalized anxiety disorder in the National Comorbidity Survey. Arch Gen Psychiatry 51:355–364, 1994

Wittchen HU, Carter RM, Pfister H, et al: Disabilities and quality of life in pure and comorbid generalized anxiety disorder and major depression in a national survey. Int Clin Psychopharmacol 15:319–328, 2000

Woodman CL, Noyes R, Black DW, et al: A 5-year follow-up study of generalized anxiety disorder and panic disorder. J Nerv Ment Dis 187:3–9, 1999

Yonkers KA, Warshaw MG, Massion AO, et al: Phenomenology and course of generalized anxiety disorder. Am J Psychiatry 168:308–313, 1996

Zatzick DF, Marmar CR, Weiss DS, et al: Posttraumatic stress disorder and functioning and quality of life outcomes in a nationally representative sample of male Vietnam veterans. Am J Psychiatry 154:1690–1695, 1997

Zlotnick C, Warshaw M, Shea MT, et al: Chronicity in posttraumatic stress disorder (PTSD) and predictors of course of comorbid PTSD in patients with anxiety disorders. J Trauma Stress 12:89–100, 1999

4

BIOLOGICAL THEORIES

Anxiety disorders are one of the best studied groups of psychiatric disorders in terms of their biological underpinnings. In the past 10 years, progress in imaging and in ligand and genetic studies have allowed us to start putting together more complete models of brain dysfunction in anxiety disorders, as well as to begin to identify common pathways the various anxiety disorders may share, such as dysregulation of the fear response to differing stimuli according to the particular disorder.

■ PANIC DISORDER

Certain pharmacologic agents have a powerful and specific capacity to induce panic attacks, in contrast to other agents that produce prominent physiological changes but fail to induce panic attacks. Similarly, admittedly terrifying situations may elicit strong fear, but not panic attacks, in those who are not vulnerable to panic attacks, whereas other seemingly much more benign situational stimuli may trigger panic attacks in those who are vulnerable. This general perspective clearly demonstrates that panic is a not a nonspecific reaction to highly distressing stimuli, but probably has a specific biological foundation, even if it might be activated through various neurochemical pathways, triggers, and circuits. A number of biological theories of panic disorder figure prominently in the literature; the evidence for and against the more promising ones is summarized here (see Table 4–1). The various theories described here should not be viewed as mutually exclusive, but rather as potentially interlocking pieces of a larger puzzle.

TABLE 4–1.	Biological models of panic disorder

Hyperreactivity of the locus coeruleus
Decreased GABA-benzodiazepine receptor complex binding
Dysregulated serotonergic modulation
HPA axis dysregulation
Hypersensitive brain stem carbon dioxide chemoreceptors
Hypersensitive conditioned fear network centered in the amygdala
Moderate genetic component

Note. GABA = gamma-aminobutyric acid; HPA = hypothalamic-pituitary-adrenal.

Sympathetic System

For many years the possibility that panic attacks are manifestations of massive discharge from the beta-adrenergic nervous system has been considered. However, elevated plasma levels of epinephrine are not a regular accompaniment of panic attacks induced in the laboratory (Liebowitz et al. 1985). Patients with spontaneous anxiety might possibly be more sensitive to the effects of isoproterenol than are subjects without psychiatric or medical disorders (Rainey et al. 1984), but the putative panicogenic effect of isoproterenol could be indirect, because isoproterenol does not cross the blood-brain barrier. Peripheral mismatch may perhaps occur between induced metabolic demands and actual physiological state and might then be conveyed to the brain stem and elicit a panic reaction (Gorman et al. 1989a). Also not supporting the beta-adrenergic hypothesis is the fact that no study has shown beta-adrenergic blockers to be effective in blocking spontaneous panic attacks. For example, intravenously administrated propranolol, in doses sufficient to achieve full peripheral beta-adrenergic blockade, is not able to block a sodium lactate–induced panic attack in patients with panic disorder (Gorman et al. 1983). Examination of various autonomic parameters seems to dispel the notion of a simple autonomic dysregulation in panic disorder (Stein and Asmundson 1994). Indeed, there does not appear to be global sympathetic activation in panic disorder patients at rest, nor even during panic attacks in some patients (Wilkinson et al. 1998).

The locus coeruleus has also been implicated in the pathogenesis of panic attacks. This nucleus is located in the pons and contains more than 50% of all noradrenergic neurons in the entire central nervous system (CNS). It sends afferent projections widely throughout the brain, including the hippocampus, amygdala, limbic system, and cerebral cortex. Electrical stimulation of the animal locus coeruleus produces a marked fear and anxiety response, whereas ablation of the animal locus coeruleus renders an animal less susceptible to a fear response in the face of threatening stimuli (Redmond 1979). In humans, drugs known to be capable of increasing locus coeruleus discharge are anxiogenic, whereas many drugs that curtail locus coeruleus firing and decrease central noradrenergic turnover are anxiolytic. For example, yohimbine challenge was reported to induce greater anxiety and a greater increase in plasma 3-methoxy-4-hydroxyphenylglycol (MHPG), a major noradrenergic metabolite, in patients with frequent panic attacks than in patients with less frequent panic attacks or healthy control subjects. Such a finding is suggestive of heightened central noradrenergic activity in panic disorder (Charney et al. 1984). The results from challenge tests with the alpha$_2$-adrenergic agonist clonidine, although difficult to interpret, have suggested noradrenergic dysregulation in panic disorder, with hypersensitivity of some and subsensitivity of other brain alpha$_2$-adrenoreceptors. Compared with the control subjects, panic disorder patients had heightened cardiovascular responses (Charney and Heninger 1986; Nutt 1989) but blunted growth hormone responses (Nutt 1989; Tancer et al. 1993) to clonidine. Dysregulated noradrenergic function, in the form of markedly elevated MHPG volatility in response to clonidine challenge, has been described in panic disorder patients, and normalizes after treatment with selective serotonin (5-hydroxytryptamine [5-HT]) reuptake inhibitors (SSRIs) (Coplan et al. 1997).

However, buspirone, which is also reported to increase locus coeruleus firing, is an anxiolytic medication and has not been reported to induce panic attacks. Medications that curtail locus coeruleus firing include clonidine, propranolol, benzodiazepines, morphine, endorphins, and tricyclic antidepressants. The medications that curtail locus coeruleus range from those that are clearly effective in blocking human panic attacks (e.g., tricyclic antidepressants) to those of more dubious efficacy (e.g., clonidine, propranolol, and standard benzodiazepines). Also, controversy exists about the relevance of animal models, and there is no consistent pattern of increased locus coeruleus discharge associated with anxiety in animals (Mason and Fibiger 1979). The locus coeruleus may be involved in arousal and response to novel stimuli rather than in anxiety (Aston-Jones et al. 1984).

GABA-Benzodiazepine System

The gamma-aminobutyric acid (GABA)–benzodiazepine receptor complex has also been implicated in the biology of panic disorder. Binding of a benzodiazepine to the benzodiazepine receptor facilitates the inhibitory action of GABA, effectively slowing neural transmission. One series of compounds, the beta-carbolines, which are inverse agonists of this receptor complex, produce an acute anxiety syndrome when administered to laboratory animals or to healthy human volunteers (Dorrow et al. 1983; Skolnick and Paul 1982). Conversely, high-potency benzodiazepines have long been known to be a highly efficacious treatment for panic disorder. The possibility is then raised that either aberrant production of an endogenous ligand or altered receptor sensitivity might occur in patients with panic disorder, interfering with proper benzodiazepine receptor function and causing their symptoms. There is some support for such a theory, although findings to date have not been consistent. One study found that panic disorder patients, compared with healthy control subjects, demonstrated less reduced saccadic eye movement velocity in response to diazepam, suggesting hyposensitivity of the benzodiazepine receptor in panic disorder (Roy-Byrne et al. 1990). The benzodiazepine antagonist flumazenil was found to be panicogenic in panic disorder patients but not in healthy control subjects, suggesting a deficiency in an endogenous anxiolytic ligand or altered benzodiazepine receptor sensitivity in panic disorder (Nutt et al. 1990). However, another study of flumazenil responses in panic disorder was negative (Strohle et al. 1999).

More recently, imaging studies have consistently revealed alterations in this system. Decreased benzodiazepine receptor binding, measured by single photon emission computed tomography (SPECT), was found in the hippocampus of panic disorder patients, and prefrontal cortex binding was also decreased in the study participants who experienced an attack during the scanning (Bremner et al. 2000). These findings could tie in neatly to the current neurocircuitry-of-fear model of panic disorder, described below, in which the amygdala, hippocampus, and prefrontal cortex play a central role in modulating conditioned fear responses. Similarly, a global decrease in benzodiazepine receptor binding has been found by positron emission tomography (PET), most prominent in the prefrontal cortex and the insula (Malizia et al. 1998). Finally, a 22% reduction in total occipital GABA levels was recently found in subjects with panic disorder, compared with control subjects (Goddard et al. 2001), as measured by 1H magnetic resonance spectroscopy.

Serotonergic System

Although the serotonergic system has not been as extensively investigated in panic disorder as other neurochemical systems, it is widely thought that it may be one of the systems that at least indirectly modulate dysregulated responses in the disorder. Indirect evidence is provided by the high efficacy of 5-HT reuptake inhibitors in treating panic disorder. It has recently been proposed that serotonergic medications may act by desensitizing the brain's fear network via projections from the raphe nuclei to the locus coeruleus, inhibiting noradrenergic activation; to the periaqueductal gray region, inhibiting freeze/flight responses; to the hypothalamus, inhibiting corticotropin-releasing factor (CRF) release; and possibly directly at the level of the amygdala, inhibiting excitatory pathways from the cortex and the thalamus (Gorman et al. 2000). A recent study of tryptophan, a 5-HT precursor, depletion found that it resulted in increased anxiety and carbon dioxide–induced panic attacks in patients with panic disorder, but not in comparison subjects (Miller et al. 2000).

Hypothalamic-Pituitary-Adrenal Axis

The hypothalamic-pituitary-adrenal (HPA) axis, which is central to an organism's response to stress, is clearly of interest in panic disorder in which a greater number of early-life stressful events, such as separations, losses, and abuse, have been described (Horesh et al. 1997; Stein et al. 1996; Tweed et al. 1989). However, HPA findings have not been consistent in panic disorder. Cortisol responses in lactate-induced panic attacks have suggested HPA axis involvement in anticipatory anxiety—as is known to occur in other anxiety and stress states—but not in the actual panic attacks (Hollander et al. 1989). There is some evidence for uncoupling of noradrenergic and HPA axis activity in panic disorder patients (Coplan et al. 1995). In a recent study, adrenocorticotropic hormone (ACTH) and cortisol responses to CRF challenge were not clearly altered in panic disorder patients compared with subjects without panic disorder (Curtis et al. 1997).

Panicogen Sodium Lactate Model

Although the panicogen sodium lactate model is not without some controversy, sodium lactate provocation of panic attacks has traditionally captured a lot of attention as an experimental model for understanding the pathogenesis of spontaneous panic attacks. Lactate-provoked panic attacks are specific to patients with prior spontaneous attacks, closely resemble the spontaneous attacks, and can be blocked by the same drugs that block natural attacks (Liebowitz et al. 1984). Cohen and White (1950) first noted that patients with neurocirculatory asthenia, a condition closely related to anxiety disorder, developed higher levels of blood lactate while exercising than did healthy control subjects. This finding stimulated Pitts and McClure (1967) to administer intravenous infusions of sodium lactate to patients with "anxiety" disorder; they found that most of the patients had an anxiety attack during infusion. The subjects all believed that these attacks were quite typical of their naturally occurring attacks. Control subjects without psychological and medical problems did not experience panic attacks during infusion.

Since the finding has been replicated on numerous occasions under proper experimental conditions, it is now a well-accepted fact that 10 mL/kg of 0.5 molar sodium lactate infused during a 20-minute period will provoke a panic attack in most patients with panic disorder but not in healthy control subjects. The mechanism, however, that may account for the observed biochemical and physiological changes (Liebowitz et al. 1985) has been the subject of much uncertainty and controversy. Theories of the mechanism have included the following: nonspecific arousal that cognitively triggers panic attacks; induction of metabolic alkalosis; hypocalcemia; alteration of the ratio of nicotinamide-adenine dinucleotide (NAD) to NADH, the reduced form of NAD (the NAD-NADH ratio); and transient intracerebral hypercapnia. Of these, transient intracerebral hypercapnia has received considerable interest and validation in recent studies and is discussed below.

Carbon Dioxide Hypersensitivity Theory

Patients with panic disorder who breathe air infused with carbon dioxide experience panic attacks almost as often as do panic disorder patients who are administered a sodium lactate infusion (Gorman et al. 1984). This finding has been consistently replicated. Similarly, sodium bicarbonate infusion provokes panic attacks in patients with panic disorder at a rate comparable to that induced by carbon dioxide inhalation (Gorman et al. 1989b). By what mechanism, then, does 5% carbon dioxide induce panic attacks? Carbon dioxide hypersensitivity may be partially explained by the findings of Svensson and colleagues, who have shown that carbon dioxide–infused air causes a reliable dose-dependent increase in locus coeruleus firing in rats (Elam et al. 1981). An alternate explanation is that patients with panic disorder might have hypersensitive brain stem carbon dioxide chemoreceptors. Indeed, during the carbon dioxide procedure, panic disorder patients who experience panic attacks while breathing 5% carbon dioxide demonstrate a much faster increase in inspiratory drive than do nonpanicking patients or normal control subjects; inspiratory drive is thought to reflect most directly the brain stem component of respiratory regulation (Gorman et al. 1988).

Such a model is of interest as it could account for the generally well established fact that hyperventilation does not cause panic attacks, whereas carbon dioxide, lactate, and bicarbonate do. Infused lactate is metabolized to bicarbonate, which is then converted in the periphery to carbon dioxide. In other words, carbon dioxide constitutes the common metabolic product of both lactate and bicarbonate. This carbon dioxide then selectively crosses the blood-brain barrier and produces transient cerebral hypercapnia. The hypercapnia then sets off the brain stem carbon dioxide chemoreceptors, leading to hyperventilation and panic attack. Thus, a "false suffocation alarm" theory of panic disorder has been formulated (Klein 1993); it proposes that patients with panic disorder are hypersensitive to carbon dioxide because they have an overly sensitive brain stem suffocation alarm system. This condition constitutes, in a sense, the opposite of the hyposensitive suffocation alarm seen in primary alveolar hypoventilation (sometimes called "Ondine's curse"), a rare illness in which persons who have the condition are at risk of suffocating in their sleep. Klein (1993) proposed that this theory of panic disorder could explain, for example, the tendency of panic attacks to occur during high–carbon dioxide states such as deep non–rapid eye movement (NREM) sleep, the premenstrual period, and sometimes relaxation—but not during childbirth, an event otherwise characterized by extreme hyperventilation and potentially catastrophic cognitions.

The carbon dioxide hypersensitivity theory may also be supported by the variety of subtle respiratory dysfunctions that appear to be associated with panic disorder, such as preexisting pulmonary disease, panic disorder patients' tendency to chronically hyperventilate, their increased variance in tidal volume during steady-state respiration, and their greater irregularities in nocturnal breathing (Papp et al. 1993; Stein et al. 1995a). There is some evidence that irregular breathing patterns are intrinsic to panic disorder patients and are not influenced by induced hyperventilation or cognitive manipulation, suggesting a brain stem rather than a higher brain level dysregulation (Abelson et al. 2001). On the other hand, Gorman and colleagues (2000) have argued that brain stem respiratory centers comprise a secondary mechanism by which panic attack symptoms relating to respiration become manifest, as one of several pathways that become activated by central excitation of the amygdala. This model of panic disorder is described below.

Neurocircuitry of Fear

A very recent model of panic disorder has been proposed that attempts to integrate neurochemical, imaging, and treatment findings in panic disorder, coupled with mostly preclinical work in the neurobiology of conditioned fear responses (Coplan and Lydiard 1998; Gorman et al. 2000). The model proposes that panic attacks are to a degree analogous to animal fear-and-avoidance responses and may be manifestations of dysregulation of the brain circuits underlying conditioned fear responses. Panic attacks are speculated to originate in an unusually sensitive fear network centered in the amygdala. Input into the amygdala is modulated by both thalamic input and prefrontal cortical projections, and amygdalar projections extend to several areas involved in various aspects of the fear response—such as the locus coeruleus and arousal, the brain stem and respiratory activation, the hypothalamus and activation of the HPA stress axis, and the cortex and cognitive interpretations. This model is thought to explain why a variety of biologically diverse agents have panicogenic properties by acting on different pathways or neurochemical systems of this network. The respiratory brain stem nucleus could not be directly triggered by such a variety of agents (Gorman et al. 2000). Thus, dysregulated "cross-talk" between the various neurotransmitter systems previously described—such as serotonergic, noradrenergic, GABAergic, CRF and others—may underlie the pathogenesis of panic disorder (Coplan and Lydiard 1998). This theory is a very comprehensive and theoretically exciting biological model of panic disorder, which, however, still needs extensive empirical validation.

Genetics

Several family and twin studies have consistently supported the presence of a moderate genetic influence in the expression of panic disorder. Crowe and colleagues (1983) found a 24.7% morbidity risk for panic disorder among the relatives of patients with panic disorder, compared with only 2.3% among healthy control subjects. Torgersen completed a study of 32 monozygotic and 53 dizygotic twins and found panic attacks to be five times more frequent in the monozygotic twins. However, the absolute concordance rate in monozygotic twins was 31%, suggesting that nongenetic factors also play an important role in the development of the disorder. Patients with occasional unexpected panic attacks may be genetically similar to patients with panic disorder, as revealed in a twin study by Torgersen and colleagues (1983) that found the best results for genetic linkage when patients with regular panic attacks were included together with patients who had only occasional panic attacks. Moderate heritability was also found in a female twin study (Kendler et al. 1993). Persons with an early onset of panic disorder appear to have a much higher familial aggregation of the disorder, possibly suggesting a stronger genetic component in a familial subtype of panic disorder, a suggestion that might better lend itself to molecular genetic studies (Goldstein et al. 1997).

Molecular genetics of panic disorders has been quite actively studied in recent years and hold promise for the future. However, a whole-genome scan in 23 panic disorder pedigrees did not yield any evidence of linkage (Knowles et al. 1998). Also, there have been several negative studies of putative genetic markers and candidate genes for panic disorder in the last decade, such as a linkage study of eight $GABA_A$ receptor genes (Crowe et al. 1997), and two studies of the 5-HT transporter gene (Deckert et al. 1997; Ishiguro et al.

1997). Some studies have yielded positive results for a variety of candidate genes, including the X-linked monoamine oxidase A gene in females (Deckert et al. 1999), the cholecystokinin gene (Wang et al. 1998), the cholecystokinin receptor gene (Kennedy et al. 1999), and the adenosine A_{2a} receptor gene (Deckert et al. 1998). These isolated genetic polymorphisms are best viewed as individual risk factors that possibly increase susceptibility to the disorder but in and of themselves are neither necessary nor sufficient for phenotypic expression.

■ GENERALIZED ANXIETY DISORDER

Although the neurobiology of generalized anxiety disorder (GAD) is among the least investigated in the anxiety disorders, advances are now being made. (See Table 4–2 for a summary of biological models of GAD.) Recent work has focused on brain circuits underlying the neurobiology of fear in animal models and in humans, and on how inherited and acquired vulnerabilities in these circuits might underlie a variety of anxiety disorders. It is speculated that alterations in the structure and function of the amygdala, which are central to fear-related behaviors, may be associated with GAD. This speculation was supported in a magnetic resonance imaging (MRI) volumetric study comparing children and adolescents with GAD with healthy comparison subjects matched for other general characteristics. The study showed those with GAD had larger right and total amygdala volumes, whereas other brain regions were comparable in size between the GAD group and the control group (DeBellis et al. 2000). The frontal cortex and medial temporal lobe are involved in controlling fear and anxiety, and there is evidence for heightened cortical activity and decreased basal ganglia activity in GAD, possibly accounting for the observed arousal and hypervigilance that occur in the disorder (Buchsbaum et al. 1987; Wu et al. 1991).

Abnormalities of the GABA-benzodiazepine receptor complex have also been implicated in GAD. The benzodiazepine receptor is linked to a receptor for the inhibitory neurotransmitter GABA.

TABLE 4–2.	Biological models of generalized anxiety disorder

Hypersensitive conditioned fear network centered in the amygdala
Abnormalities of the GABA-benzodiazepine receptor
Noradrenergic activation
Serotonergic dysregulation
Modest genetic component

Note. GABA = gamma-aminobutyric acid.

The beta-carbolines, which are inverse agonists of this receptor complex, produce an acute anxiety syndrome when administered to laboratory animals or to healthy human volunteers (Dorrow et al. 1983; Skolnick and Paul 1982). Conversely, benzodiazepines are well established as an efficacious treatment of GAD. Persons with GAD were found to have decreased benzodiazepine receptor density in peripheral blood cells, as well as decreased transcriptional messenger ribonucleic acid (mRNA) encoding for the receptor— both of these return to normal values with treatment and reduction in anxiety levels (Ferrarese et al. 1990; Rocca et al. 1998). Similarly, benzodiazepine receptor binding has been found to be greatly decreased in the left temporal lobe of GAD patients compared with psychologically healthy control subjects (Tiihonen et al. 1997).

Objective sleep disturbances have been described in GAD patients on polysomnography and electroencephalographic mapping, again concordant with CNS hypervigilance and hyperarousal (Saletu et al. 1997). Evidence for noradrenergic dysregulation has yielded mixed results. Abelson and colleagues reported a blunted growth hormone response to clonidine in GAD patients compared with responses in control subjects without psychological or medical problems (Abelson et al. 1991). Plasma norepinephrine and its metabolite were found to be elevated, and alpha$_2$-adrenoreceptors decreased, in GAD patients compared with psychologically and medically healthy control subjects (Sevy et al. 1989). Other studies of the noradrenergic system have been negative (Mathew et al. 1981). There is also some evidence of serotonergic dysregulation in persons with GAD, such as heightened anxiety responses to the partial 5-HT agonist *m*-chlorophenylpiperazine (m-CPP), compared to control subjects (Germine et al. 1992). Indirect support is also derived from the efficacy of buspirone, a $5-HT_1$ agonist, and nefazodone, a $5-HT_2$ antagonist, in treating GAD. Patients with GAD do not show heightened sensitivity to 5% carbon dioxide inhalation, as do those with panic disorder, supporting the conceptualization of the disorders as two discrete disorders (Perna et al. 1999).

There appears to be a genetic component to GAD, albeit relatively modest. A 19.5% morbidity risk for GAD was found among relatives of GAD patients compared with 3.5% in psychologically and medically healthy control relatives; this risk may have represent an overestimate, because the GAD in the relatives was less chronic, less severe, or less likely to be treated than in the probands (Noyes et al. 1987). In the Torgersen (1983) study of 32 monozygotic and 53 dizygotic twins, no difference was found in the monozygotic-dizygotic concordance rate for GAD. However, Kendler and colleagues, studying GAD in female twins, determined that the familial component of the disorder was almost entirely genetic, with a modest heritability of about 30% (Kendler et al. 1992a). There have been minimal molecular genetic studies of GAD to date—which require replication—that have suggested associations to polymorphisms of the dopamine D_2 receptor gene (Peroutka et al. 1998), the 5-HT transporter gene (Ohara et al. 1999), and the dopamine transporter gene (Rowe et al. 1998).

■ SOCIAL PHOBIA

Neurochemistry

Neurochemical studies of social phobia have not been as systematic or consistently replicated as those in panic disorder, but they have to date implicated a number of neurotransmitter systems, including the noradrenergic, GABAergic, dopaminergic, and serotonergic. Patients with social phobia were found to exhibit a blunted growth hormone response to clonidine challenge, implicating noradrenergic dysfunction similar to that of panic disorder patients (Tancer et al. 1993). However, this finding was not replicated in a subsequent study (Tancer et al. 1994). Patients with social phobia also show evidence of altered autonomic responsivity, such as an exaggerated response to the Valsalva maneuver compared with controls without psychological and medical problems (Stein et al. 1994). GABA-benzodiazepine receptor involvement is unclear. One study found that the benzodiazepine antagonist flumazenil did not induce a greater surge in anxiety in social phobia compared with control subjects (Coupland et al. 2000). However, another study showed greatly decreased peripheral benzodiazepine receptor density in patients with generalized social phobia compared with a medically and psychologically healthy group (Johnson et al. 1998). Despite the now documented efficacy of 5-HT reuptake inhibitors in treating social phobia, little is directly known about serotonergic involvement in the disorder. One study found increased cortisol response to fenfluramine, suggestive of altered serotonergic sensitivity (Tancer et al. 1994). However, social phobia patients in other studies showed no evidence of altered 5-HT reuptake sites in platelets (Stein et al. 1995b), and no abnormality in the prolactin response to m-CPP (Hollander et al. 1998). Two studies found normal basal functioning of the HPA axis in social phobia, as measured by basal cortisol levels and the dexamethasone suppression test (Uhde et al. 1994), but HPA studies under social stress could be more telling. There is also evidence that social phobia may be associated with a decreased central dopaminergic tone, such as indirect evidence of social phobia triggered by dopamine blocking agents (Mikkelson et al. 1981) or treatment of social anxiety with the dopamine reuptake inhibitor bupropion (Emmanuel et al. 1991). Persons with comorbid panic disorder and social phobia have been found to have decreased levels of the dopamine metabolite homovanillic acid in the cerebrospinal fluid (CSF) (Johnson et al. 1994). Finally, in more definitive recent studies, social phobia was associated with a 20% decrease in dopamine transporter site density in the striatum by SPECT (Tiihonen et al. 1997) and, similarly, with lowered dopamine D_2 receptor binding potential (Schneier et al. 2000), although these findings need to be replicated.

Imaging Studies

The neuroimaging of social phobia is still in its infancy. One structural imaging study found no volumetric differences in patients with social phobia compared to fa psychologically healthy control group (Potts et al. 1994), and another found no differences in regional blood flow by SPECT with subjects in a basal resting state (Stein and Leslie 1996). However, provocation paradigms that evoke social anxiety symptoms during imaging might be expected to have a higher yield in revealing dysfunctional brain circuits in social phobia, and some interesting preliminary findings have been reported in the very few studies of this sort. In one small study, persons with social phobia, as compared to medically and psychologically healthy control subjects, demonstrated a selective higher activation in the amygdala (a center for the emotional processing of fearfulness) in response to emotionally neutral faces during functional magnetic resonance imaging (fMRI) (Birbaumer et al. 1998). In a PET study that used social-anxiety–provoking scripts, individuals with social phobia showed greater blood flow in the anterior cingulate, the dorsolateral prefrontal cortex, the orbitofrontal cortex, and the insula—areas involved in emotional processing; however, the amygdala was relatively deactivated (Bell et al. 1999). A SPECT study of social phobia patients who underwent imaging before and after treatment with an SSRI showed higher baseline activity in the left temporal cortex and left midfrontal regions in non-responders compared with responders (Van der Linden et al. 2000). A similar model to that described in panic disorder, involving faulty conditioned fear responses, has also been implicated in social phobia as well as other anxiety disorders, each to its specific triggers. Along these lines, one study found signal decreases in the amygdala and hippocampus in participants without medical or psychological problems when they were presented with the conditioned stimulus of a neutral face associated with an unconditioned stimulus, whereas patients with social phobia exhibited opposite increased activations in both regions (Schneider et al. 1999).

Genetics

A strong familial risk for social phobia has been identified and is believed to be partly heritable and partly environmental. First-degree relatives of probands with generalized social phobia have an approximately 10-fold higher risk for generalized social phobia or avoidant personality disorder (Stein et al. 1998a). One twin study did not support a genetic component to social phobia and specific phobia, in contrast to panic disorder, GAD, and posttraumatic stress disorder, suggesting environmental causation (Skre et al. 1993). However, in another study of phobias in twins, Kendler and his group determined that the familial aggregation of phobias was mostly accounted for by genetic factors, with a modest heritability of 30%–40%, depending on the particular phobia (Kendler et al. 1992b). Environmental factors also played a significant role in the development of phobic disorders. An adolescent female twin study estimated the heritability of social phobia to be 28%, with strong evidence for shared genetic vulnerability between social phobia and major depression (Nelson et al. 2000).

Behavioral inhibition, which is believed to be largely heritable and becomes manifest and fixed in early childhood (Kagan et al. 1987), is thought to be one of the substrates on which social phobia might develop; however, behavioral inhibition alone cannot trigger the disorder. Behavioral inhibition identified in toddlers has been found, prospectively, to be a strong predictor of social anxiety in adolescence (Schwartz et al. 1999). Similarly, behavioral inhibition, in the form of both social avoidance and fearfulness in early high school, prospectively predicted the onset of social phobia four years later (Hayward et al. 1998). Cross-sectionally, a specific association has been found between childhood shyness and maternal social phobia as opposed to other anxiety disorders (Cooper and Eke 1999).

There are essentially no genetic molecular studies in social phobia. One report found no linkage to the 5-HT transporter or 5-HT$_{2A}$ receptor gene in generalized social phobia (Stein et al. 1998b). Biological models of social phobia are summarized in Table 4–3.

TABLE 4–3.   **Biological models of social phobia**

Abnormalities of the GABA-benzodiazepine receptor
Hypersensitive conditioned fear network centered in the amygdala
Noradrenergic activation
Decreased dopaminergic tone
Modest genetic component

Note.   GABA = gamma-aminobutyric acid.

■ SPECIFIC PHOBIA

Some interesting recent hypotheses about the origin of phobias have resulted from integration of ethological, biological, and learning theory approaches. Fyer et al. (1990) found high familial transmission for specific phobias, with a roughly threefold risk for first-degree relatives of affected persons; there was no increased risk for other comorbid phobic or anxiety disorders. One twin study did not support a genetic component to specific phobias, suggesting environmental causation (Skre et al. 1993). However, in a large study of phobias in twins, Kendler and his group determined that the familial aggregation of phobias was mostly accounted for by genetic factors, with a modest heritability of 30%–40%, depending on the particular phobia (Kendler et al. 1992b). Environmental factors also played a significant role in the development of phobic disorders.

The neurobiology of specific phobias has barely been studied. Two studies examining response to carbon dioxide inhalation in persons with specific phobia found 1) no differences between the subjects with phobia and subjects without psychological and medical problems and 2) no hypersensitivity to carbon dioxide, as is found in patients with panic disorder (Antony et al. 1997; Verburg et al. 1994). Brain imaging studies in specific phobia are few and inconclusive. One showed negative findings during exposure to the phobic stimulus (Mountz et al. 1989), whereas two other studies showed activation of the visual associative cortex (Fredrikson et al. 1993) and of the somatosensory cortex (Rauch et al. 1995), suggesting that visual and tactile imagery are one component of the phobic response; findings regarding limbic activation appear equivocal.

The brain circuits mediating conditioned fear have recently been proposed as central to the pathogenesis of a number of anxiety disorders, including specific phobia, although data are extremely limited for this disorder. Such a model is attractive in that it may account for the occurrence of such a highly fearful response to the conditioned phobic stimulus without hippocampal or cortically based knowledge or memory of why there is such fear. Studies exposing specific phobia subjects to masked stimuli (i.e., very brief stimuli that can only be perceived implicitly) have lent partial support to the notion that phobic stimuli, even when not consciously registered, can elicit a subjective or objectively measured fearful response (Ohman and Soares 1994; Van Den Hout et al. 1997).

■ OBSESSIVE-COMPULSIVE DISORDER

Although obsessive-compulsive disorder (OCD) was once viewed as having a psychological etiology, a wealth of biological findings that have emerged over the past 15 years have rendered OCD one of the most elegantly elaborated psychiatric disorders from a biological standpoint. The association of OCD with a variety of neurological conditions or more subtle neurologic findings has been known for some time. Such findings include the onset of OCD following head trauma (McKeon et al. 1984) or von Economo disease (Schilder 1938); a high incidence of neurological premorbid illnesses in OCD (Grimshaw 1964); an association of OCD with birth trauma (Capstick and Seldrup 1977); abnormalities on the electroencephalogram (Pacella et al. 1944); auditory evoked potentials (Ciesielski et al. 1981; Towey et al. 1990); ventricular brain ratio on computed tomography (Behar et al. 1984); an association with diabetes insipidus (Barton 1965); and the presence of significantly more neurological soft signs in OCD patients compared with healthy control subjects (Hollander et al. 1990). Basal ganglia abnormalities were particularly suspected in the pathogenesis of

OCD, given that OCD is closely associated with Tourette syndrome (Nee et al. 1982; Pauls et al. 1986), in which basal ganglia dysfunction results in abnormal involuntary movements, as well as with Sydenham chorea, another disorder of the basal ganglia (Barton 1965; Swedo et al. 1989a). Neuropsychological findings in OCD have also been of some interest, although not always consistent, and have suggested abnormalities in memory, memory confidence, trial-and-error learning, and processing speed (Christensen et al. 1992; Galderisi et al. 1996; McNally and Kohlbeck 1993; Otto 1992; Rubenstein et al. 1993). Table 4–4 summarizes biological perspectives on OCD, which are described below.

TABLE 4–4.   **Biological models of obsessive-compulsive disorder**

Serotonergic dysregulation
Additional dopaminergic dysregulation, at least in subgroup of patients
Neuropeptide abnormalities (oxytocin, vasopressin, somatostatin)
Hyperactive orbitofrontal–limbic–basal-ganglia circuitry
Autoimmune streptococcal-related component in some persons
Genetic component; possible polymorphisms of the COMT, 5-HT
    transporter, and 5-HT_{1D} receptor genes

Note.   COMT = catechol-O-methyltransferase; 5-HT = serotonin.

Serotonergic System

The neurochemistry of OCD has been extensively elaborated in the past two decades. 5-HT is implicated in mediating impulsivity, suicidality, aggression, anxiety, social dominance, and learning. Despite some conflicting and nonreplicated data, extensive research has now clearly implicated the serotonergic system in the pathogenesis of OCD. Considerable indirect evidence supporting the role of 5-HT in OCD stems from the well-documented antiobsessional effects of potent 5-HT reuptake inhibitors such as clomipramine and the SSRIs, in contrast to the ineffectiveness of noradrenergic antidepressants such as desipramine. Furthermore, reduction of OCD symptoms during clomipramine treatment was shown to correlate with a decrease in platelet 5-HT level (Flament et al. 1987) and in CSF 5-hydroxyindoleacetic acid (5-HIAA) (Altemus et al. 1992; Swedo et al. 1992; Thorén et al. 1980). Although one study reported higher CSF 5-HIAA in untreated OCD patients compared with healthy control subjects (Insel et al. 1985), this finding has not been replicated (Thorén et al. 1980).

The use of pharmacologic challenge agents to stimulate or block 5-HT receptors has also proved a fruitful technique in elucidating the neurochemistry of OCD. Oral m-CPP, a partial 5-HT agonist, was found to transiently exacerbate obsessive-compulsive symptoms in a subgroup of OCD patients (Hollander et al. 1992; Zohar et al. 1987). Studies with intravenous m-CPP showed mixed results (Charney et al. 1988; Pigott et al. 1993). After treatment of OCD with 5-HT reuptake blockers such as clomipramine or fluoxetine, m-CPP challenge no longer induced exacerbation of symptoms (Hollander et al. 1991a; Zohar et al. 1988). A blunted prolactin response to m-CPP challenge has also been found in OCD patients by some investigators (Charney et al. 1988; Hollander et al. 1992) but not others (Zohar et al. 1987). Similarly blunted prolactin responses in OCD have been induced with the 5-HT agonist MK-212 (Bastani et al. 1990). Other 5-HT agonists, such as tryptophan, fenfluramine and ipsapirone, or antagonists such as metergoline, have not been shown to induce consistent behavioral or neuroendocrine response abnormalities in patients with OCD (Benkelfat et al. 1989; Charney et al. 1988; Hewlett et al. 1992; Hollander et al. 1992; Lesch et al. 1991; McBride et al. 1992; Zohar et al. 1987).

In summary, all studies taken together suggest that serotonergic dysregulation in OCD is complex and probably involves variations in receptor function according to brain region and receptor subtypes. Thus global hyperactivity or hypoactivity of the serotonergic system in OCD is a simplistic formulation. The m-CPP findings may suggest hypersensitivity of the 5-HT receptors mediating obsessive-compulsive behaviors, but also hyporesponsivity of the hypothalamic 5-HT receptors mediating prolactin secretion (Hollander et al. 1992).

Other Neurochemical Systems

It does not appear that serotonergic dysregulation alone can fully explain the neurochemistry of OCD. It is also possible that the serotonergic system may, in part, be modulating or compensating for other dysfunctional neurotransmitter systems or neuromodulators. Various neuropeptide abnormalities have started to be elucidated in the past decade. Abnormalities in CSF vasopressin (Altemus et al. 1992; Swedo et al. 1992), CSF somatostatin (Altemus et al. 1993), and CSF oxytocin (Leckman et al. 1994) have been implicated in OCD. With clomipramine treatment, CSF levels of vasopressin and somatostatin tend to decrease while oxytocin increases (Altemus et al. 1994). All these neuropeptides may be implicated in arousal, memory, and the acquisition and maintenance of conditioned perseverative behaviors.

The alpha$_2$-adrenergic agonist clonidine has been reported to induce a transient improvement in OCD symptoms when administered to patients intravenously (Hollander et al. 1991b) or orally (Knesevich 1982), although other noradrenergic challenge findings have been negative (Lucey et al. 1992).

Dopaminergic dysregulation has been variously implicated in OCD (Goodman et al. 1990) through the association between OCD and Tourette syndrome; reports of exacerbation of obsessive-compulsive symptoms with chronic stimulants; an association between higher pretreatment CSF homovanillic acid and good treatment outcome (Swedo et al. 1992); blunted growth hormone response to the dopamine agonist apomorphine (Brambilla et al. 1997); and use of dopamine blockers to augment partial treatment response with 5-HT reuptake blockers (McDougle et al. 1990).

Imaging and the Orbitofrontal–Limbic–Basal Ganglia Circuitry

Recent neuroimaging techniques have permitted a more sophisticated and elaborate elucidation of the functional anatomy underpinning OCD. In particular, orbitofrontal–limbic–basal ganglia circuits have been implicated in numerous studies. Baxter et al. (1987), using PET, compared OCD patients and control subjects without a mental disorder and found higher metabolic rates in the orbitofrontal gyri and caudate nuclei in patients with OCD. Similarly, Swedo and her group found higher metabolic activity in the orbitofrontal and cingulate regions in persons with OCD (Swedo et al. 1989b). Flor-Henry (1983) hypothesized that "the fundamental symptomatology of obsessions is due to a defect in neural inhibition of dominant frontal systems, leading to the inability to inhibit unwanted verbal-ideational mental representations and their corresponding motor sequences" (p. 309). It has been suggested that the severity of obsessive urges correlates with orbitofrontal and basal ganglia activity, whereas the accompanying anxiety is reflected by activity in the hippocampus and cingulate cortex (McGuire et al. 1994). With fMRI, it has been possible to demonstrate that during the behavioral provocation of symptoms in OCD patients, significant increases in relative blood flow occur in "real" time in the caudate, cingulate cortex, and orbitofrontal cortex relative to the resting state (Adler et al. 2000; Breiter et al. 1996; Rauch et al. 1994). In addition, higher-resolution MRI techniques have revealed abnormal volumes of a variety of brain regions in OCD, including reduced orbitofrontal and amygdala volumes (Szeszko et al. 1999), smaller basal ganglia (Rosenberg et al. 1997), and enlarged thalamus (Gilbert et al. 2000).

Of great interest are a number of studies that have now been conducted, demonstrating not only functional but also structural brain changes after a variety of treatments for OCD. After treatment of the OCD with 5-HT reuptake blockers or with behavior therapy, hyperactivity decreases in the caudate, in the orbitofrontal lobes, and in the cingulate cortex in those patients who have good treatment responses (Baxter et al. 1992; Benkelfat et al. 1990; Perani et al. 1995; Swedo et al. 1992). Also, after successful behavioral treatment, the correlations in brain activity between the orbital gyri and the caudate nucleus decrease significantly, suggesting a decoupling of malfunctioning brain circuits (Schwartz et al. 1996). In children with OCD, a decrease in initially abnormally large thalamic size has been imaged with successful response to paroxetine treatment (Gilbert et al. 2000). This finding was not replicated in children in response to cognitive behavioral therapy (Rosenberg et al. 2000a). Magnetic resonance spectroscopy has also revealed a decrease in initially elevated caudate glutamate concentration in children with OCD after successful paroxetine treatment (Rosenberg et al. 2000b).

Neuroethological Model

A neuroethological model of OCD has been proposed by Rapoport, Swedo, Cheslow, and colleagues (Swedo 1989; Wise and Rapoport 1989), based on the hypothesized orbitofrontal–limbic–basal ganglia dysfunction. The basal ganglia act as a gating station that filters input from the orbitofrontal and the cingulate cortex and mediates the execution of motor patterns. Obsessions and compulsions are conceptualized as species-specific fixed action patterns that are normally adaptive but that in OCD become inappropriately released, repetitive, and excessive. This process could be due to a heightened internal drive state or an increased responsivity to external releasers. For example, OCD behaviors such as excessive washing or saving may be dysregulated manifestations of normal grooming or hoarding behaviors. Studies documenting significant volumetric brain abnormalities in children with OCD who have not been treated for the disorder suggest that a developmentally mediated dysplasia of the ventral prefrontal-striatal circuitry may underlie OCD (Rosenberg and Keshavan 1998).

Autoimmune Processes

A certain form of OCD with childhood onset is believed to be related to an autoimmune process secondary to streptococcal infection. In children with this form of OCD, enlarged basal ganglia have been found on MRI, a finding consistent with an autoimmune process (Giedd et al. 2000). A particular B lymphocyte antigen, which can be identified by the monoclonal antibody D8/17, is expressed in nearly all patients with rheumatic fever and is thought to be a trait marker for susceptibility to group A streptococcal infection complications. Children with OCD and without a history of rheumatic fever or Sydenham chorea were found to have significantly greater B-cell D8/17 expression than control children, suggesting that D8/17 may serve as a marker for susceptibility to childhood-onset OCD (Murphy et al. 1997).

Genetics

Twin and family studies found a greater degree of concordance for OCD (defined broadly to include obsessional features) among monozygotic twins compared with dizygotic twins (Carey and Gottesman 1981), suggesting that some predisposition to obsessional behavior is inherited. There have been no studies of OCD in adopted children or monozygotic twins raised apart. Studies of first-degree relatives of OCD patients show a higher-than-expected incidence of a variety of psychiatric disorders, including obsessive-compulsive symptoms, anxiety disorders, and depression (Black et al. 1992; Carey and Gottesman 1981; Rapoport et al. 1981). Family studies suggest a genetic link between OCD and Tourette syndrome (Nee et al. 1982). A recent large family study found that OCD was about fourfold more common in relatives of OCD probands than in control relatives, and the finding was more robust for obsessions. Interestingly, age at onset of OCD in probands was very strongly related to familiality; no OCD was detected in relatives of probands with onset after age 18 (Nestadt et al. 2000a). This study suggests, as does a similar one of panic disorder, that there may exist a more strongly familial subtype of OCD with earlier age at onset. Family studies have also shown that OCD spectrum disorders, such as body dysmorphic disorder, hypochondriasis, eating disorder, and grooming conditions occur more frequently than expected in the relatives of those with OCD (Bienvenu et al. 2000).

In the past few years, the molecular genetics of OCD, still in its infancy, has been the subject of investigation. Segregation analyses have provided strong support for a single major gene involvement in OCD (Alsobrook et al. 1999; Nestadt et al. 2000b), but should this be so, the major gene has not been identified to date. A functional polymorphism of the catechol O-methyltransferase (COMT) gene with low enzymatic activity was initially implicated in a recessive manner in OCD (Karayiorgou et al. 1997, 1999), but that finding has not been consistently replicated (Schindler et al. 2000). Polymorphisms in genes related to 5-HT and dopamine transmission—such as the tryptophan hydroxylase gene, the 5-HT_{2A} receptor gene, the 5-HT_{2C} receptor gene, the 5-HT transporter gene, the dopamine D_4 receptor gene, and the dopamine transporter gene—were not shown to be associated with OCD in a study by Frisch and associates (Frisch et al. 2000). Similarly, no association was shown to mutations of the 5-HT_{2B} receptor gene (Kim et al. 2000), the tryptophan hydroxylase gene (Han et al. 1999), and the 5-HT_{2C} receptor gene (Cavallini et al. 1998). Findings regarding the 5-HT transporter gene have been both positive (Bengel et al. 1999) and negative (Billet et al. 1997). However, a polymorphism of the 5-HT_{1D} receptor gene has also been implicated (Mundo et al. 2000). In summary, then, most molecular research to date has focused on 5-HT–related gene research, which has not yielded clear and replicable findings, but is an area of active research.

■ POSTTRAUMATIC STRESS DISORDER

More than a century ago, Janet described the breakdown in normal adaptation, information processing, and action that can result from overwhelming trauma and noted the automatic emotional and physical overreaction that occurs with reexposure (van der Kolk and van der Hart 1989). Freud (1926/1959) implicated a biological basis in posttraumatic symptoms, in the form of a physical fixation to the trauma. Pavlov (1927/1960) demonstrated chronic change in autonomic nervous system activity level in response to repeated traumatic exposure. Kardiner (1959) comprehensively described the phenomenology of war traumatic neurosis, identifying five cardinal features: 1) persistence of startle response, 2) fixation on the trauma, 3) atypical dream life, 4) explosive outbursts, and 5) overall constriction of the personality. He labeled this condition a *physioneurosis*, implying an interaction of psychological and biological processes, thus providing a forerunner of current psycho-biological models of posttraumatic stress disorder (PTSD). Table 4–5 summarizes current biological perspectives on PTSD described below.

TABLE 4–5.	**Biological models of posttraumatic stress disorder**

Heightened physiologic responses to traumatic stimuli
Noradrenergic activation
Highly sensitized HPA axis
Endogenous opioid dysregulation
Dysregulated serotonergic modulation
Hippocampal toxicity, decreased volumes
Limbic hyperactivity (amygdala, cingulate) and cortical hyporesponsivity
   (prefrontal, Broca's area) to traumatic stimuli

Note.   HPA = hypothalamic-pituitary-adrenal

Sympathetic System

Neurobiological response to acute stress involves the release of various stress hormones (e.g., heightened secretion of catecholamines and cortisol) that allows the organism to respond adaptively. When PTSD develops under severe or repeated trauma, the stress response becomes dysregulated, and chronic autonomic hyperactivity sets in. This process manifests itself in the "positive" symptoms of PTSD, such as hyperarousal and intrusive symptoms. A wide range of data supports this hypothesis. In patients with PTSD, heightened autonomic physiological responses to stressful stimuli—such as blood pressure, heart rate, respiration rate, galvanic skin response, and electromyographic activity—have been consistently documented (Kolb 1987; Pitman et al. 1987).

   The noradrenergic system, originating in the locus coeruleus, regulates arousal. Animals exposed to inescapable shock initially show evidence of increased turnover of norepinephrine, with subsequent depletion of central norepinephrine (Anisman et al. 1980). Animals that have experienced previous inescapable shock are more sensitive to norepinephrine depletion. Long-standing increases in the urinary catecholamines norepinephrine and epinephrine have been found in PTSD patients (Kosten et al. 1987; Spivak et al. 1999), as well as elevated plasma norepinephrine (Spivak et al. 1999). Agents that stimulate the arousal system, such as lactate (Rainey et al. 1987) and yohimbine (Southwick et al. 1993, 1997) induce flashbacks and increases in core PTSD symptoms. Clinical improvement in intrusive recollections and hyperarousal during treatment with adrenergic blocking agents such as clonidine or propranolol also suggests adrenergic hyperactivity (Kolb et al. 1984). A decrease in the number and sensitivity of alpha$_2$-adrenergic receptors, possibly as a consequence of chronic noradrenergic hyperactivity, has been reported in PTSD (Perry et al. 1987). Downregulation of the alpha$_2$-adrenergic receptor is also supported by a case report of a PTSD patient with a blunted growth hormone response to clonidine, which normalized after behavioral treatment (Hansenne et al. 1991).

Serotonergic System

The serotonergic system has also been implicated in the symptomatology of PTSD (van der Kolk and Saporta 1991). The septohippocampal brain system contains serotonergic pathways and mediates behavioral inhibition and constraint. The role of serotonergic deficit in impulsive aggression has been studied extensively. In animals, repeated inescapable shock can lead to 5-HT depletion. Thus, the irritability and outbursts seen in patients with PTSD may be related to serotonergic deficit. The partial 5-HT agonist m-CPP induces an increase in PTSD symptoms suggestive of a compensatory sensitization of the serotonergic system, and, interestingly, subjects exhibiting this response appear to be a separate subgroup of PTSD subjects from the ones exhibiting noradrenergic sensitization (Southwick et al. 1997). Decreased plasma 5-HT levels have been found in PTSD (Spivak et al. 1999). A blunted prolactin response to fenfluramine challenge is also supportive of central serotonergic dysregulation in PTSD (Davis et al. 1999). The known efficacy of

SSRIs in treating PTSD is also indirectly supportive of dysregulated serotonergic modulation.

The Hypothalamic-Pituitary-Adrenal Axis

A number of findings in PTSD have implicated a chronic dysregulation of HPA axis functioning that is highly characteristic of PTSD and distinct from that seen in other psychiatric disorders such as depression. The findings include elevated CSF corticotropin-releasing hormone (Baker et al. 1999; Bremner et al. 1997a), low urinary cortisol (Mason et al. 1986), an elevated urinary norepinephrine-cortisol ratio (Mason et al. 1988), blunted ACTH response to CRF (Smith et al. 1989), enhanced suppression of cortisol following dexamethasone administration, and a decrease in the number of lymphocyte glucocorticoid receptors. All these findings are consistent with a model of a highly sensitized HPA axis that is hyperresponsive to stress and the effects of cortisol (Yehuda et al. 1993, 1995).

Endogenous Opioid System

In the past, affective numbing was understood primarily as a psychological defense against overwhelming emotional pain, but recent research has suggested a biological component to the "negative" symptoms of PTSD. Van der Kolk and his group proposed that animal models of inescapable shock might parallel the development of PTSD in humans (van der Kolk et al. 1984). Animals prevented from escaping from severe stress develop a syndrome of learned helplessness (Maier and Seligman 1976) that resembles the symptoms of constricted affect, withdrawal, amotivation, and decline in functioning associated with PTSD. Animals exposed to prolonged or repeated inescapable stress develop analgesia, which appears to be mediated by release of endogenous opiates and which is blocked by the opiate antagonist naloxone (Kelly 1982; Maier et al. 1980). Similarly, it is suggested that in humans who have sustained prolonged or repeated trauma, endogenous opiates are readily released with any stimulus that is reminiscent of the original trauma, leading to analgesia and psychic numbing (van der Kolk et al. 1984).

Pitman and his group compared pain intensity to thermal stimuli in Vietnam veterans with PTSD and veterans without PTSD who were watching a war videotape (Pitman et al. 1990). PTSD patients, but not the subjects without PTSD, experienced a 30% analgesia in response to viewing the tape when pretreated with a placebo injection; this analgesia was eliminated with naloxone pretreatment. On the basis of such findings, the concept of trauma addiction has been proposed (van der Kolk et al. 1984). After a transient opioid burst on reexposure to traumatic stimuli, accompanied by a subjective sense of calm and control, opiate withdrawal may set in. This withdrawal may then contribute to the hyperarousal symptoms of PTSD, leading the affected person to a vicious circle of traumatic reexposures in order to gain transient symptomatic relief. The noradrenergic and opiatergic systems of the brain interact and may serve reciprocal functions. Clonidine, an alpha$_2$-adrenergic agonist, has been shown to suppress opiate withdrawal symptoms in opiate addiction (Gold et al. 1980). Open treatment with clonidine in Vietnam veterans with PTSD demonstrated substantial decreases in hyperreactivity (Kolb et al. 1984).

Imaging Studies

A number of neuroimaging findings in PTSD, both structural and functional, have begun to draw a model suggestive of limbic sensitization and diminished cortical inhibition in PTSD, with specific dysfunction in brain areas involved in memory, emotion, and visuospatial processing (Bremner et al. 1999). Functional deficits in verbal memory have been correlated with a decreased hippocampal volume, as seen on MRI, in persons with combat-related PTSD (Bremner et al. 1995). Similarly, a decrease in hippocampal volume has been found in adult survivors of childhood abuse (Bremner et al. 1997b). PET with PTSD-symptom provocation, using audiotaped traumatic scripts, showed activation of the right limbic and paralimbic systems and of the visual cortex (Rauch et al. 1996). PET during auditory exposure to traumatic scripts has shown that abuse memories are associated with decreased blood flow in the medial prefrontal cortex, hippocampus, and visual association cortex (Bremner et al. 1999b). When mental images of combat-related pictures are generated by veterans with PTSD, blood flow increases in the amygdala and anterior cingulate and decreases in Broca's area. These patterns may relate to the nonverbal emotional visual imagery involved in reexperiencing PTSD symptoms (Shin et al. 1997). Enhanced amygdala responses to general negative stimuli, not specifically related to trauma, have been found in PTSD; these appear to be dissociated from higher cortical influences (Rauch et al. 2000). Indeed, exposure of PTSD subjects to traumatic stimuli results in decreased blood flow in the medial prefrontal cortex, an area responsible for the regulation of emotional response via inhibition of the amygdala (Bremner et al. 1999). There is evidence, based on case reports, that successful treatment of PTSD with eye movement desensitization and Reprocessing (EMDR) may result not in reduced limbic activity, but rather in increased cingulate and prefrontal activity, which enhances the ability to differentiate real threat (Levin et al. 1999).

Genetics

A large study of Vietnam veteran twins found that genetic factors accounted for 13%–34% of the variance in liability to the various PTSD symptom clusters, whereas no etiologic role was found for shared environment (True et al. 1993). Molecular genetic studies of PTSD are very few. An initial study found an association with a polymorphism of the dopamine D_2 receptor (Comings et al. 1996), not replicated later (Gelernter et al. 1999).

■ REFERENCES

Abelson JL, Glitz D, Cameron OG, et al: Blunted growth hormone response to clonidine in patients with generalized anxiety disorder. Arch Gen Psychiatry 48:157–162, 1991

Abelson JL, Weg JG, Nesse RM, et al: Persistent respiratory irregularity in patients with panic disorder. Biol Psychiatry 49:588–595, 2001

Adler CM, McDonough-Ryan P, Sax KW, et al: fMRI of neuronal activation with symptom provocation in unmedicated patients with obsessive compulsive disorder. J Psychiatr Res 34:317–324, 2000

Alsobrook JP II, Leckman JF, Goodman WK, et al: Segregation analysis of obsessive-compulsive disorder using symptom-based factor scores. Am J Med Genet 88:669–675, 1999

Altemus M, Pigott T, Kalogeras KT, et al: Abnormalities in the regulation of vasopressin and corticotropin releasing factor secretion in obsessive-compulsive disorder. Arch Gen Psychiatry 49:9–20, 1992

Altemus M, Pigott T, L'Heureux F, et al: CSF somatostatin in obsessive-compulsive disorder. Am J Psychiatry 150:460–464, 1993

Altemus M, Swedo SE, Leonard HL, et al: Changes in cerebrospinal fluid neurochemistry during treatment of obsessive-compulsive disorder with clomipramine. Arch Gen Psychiatry 51:794–803, 1994

Anisman HL, Pizzino A, Sklar LS: Coping with stress, norepinephrine depletion and escape performance. Brain Res 191:583–588, 1980

Antony MM, Brown TA, Barlow DH: Response to hyperventilation and 5.5% CO_2 inhalation of subjects with types of specific phobia, panic disorder, or no mental disorder. Am J Psychiatry 154(8):1089–1095, 1997

Aston-Jones SL, Foote FE, Bloom FE: Norepinephrine, in Frontiers of Clinical Neuroscience, Vol 2. Edited by Ziegler MG, Lake CR. Baltimore, MD, Williams & Wilkins, 1984, pp 92–116

Baker DG, West SA, Nicholson WE, et al: Serial CSF corticotropin-releasing hormone levels and adrenocortical activity in combat veterans with posttraumatic stress disorder. Am J Psychiatry 156:585–588, 1999

Barton R: Diabetes insipidus and obsessional neurosis: a syndrome. Lancet 1:133–135, 1965

Bastani B, Nash JF, Meltzer HY: Prolactin and cortisol responses to MK-212, a serotonin agonist, in obsessive-compulsive disorder. Arch Gen Psychiatry 47:833–839, 1990

Baxter LR Jr, Phelps ME, Mazziotta JC, et al: Local cerebral glucose metabolic rates in obsessive-compulsive disorder: a comparison with rates in unipolar depression and in normal controls. Arch Gen Psychiatry 44:211–218, 1987

Baxter LR Jr, Schwartz JM, Bergman KS, et al: Caudate glucose metabolic rate changes with both drug and behavior therapy for obsessive-compulsive disorder. Arch Gen Psychiatry 49:681–689, 1992

Behar D, Rapoport JL, Berg CJ, et al: Computerized tomography and neuropsychological test measures in adolescents with obsessive-compulsive disorder. Am J Psychiatry 141:363–369, 1984

Bell CJ, Malizia AL, Nutt DJ: The neurobiology of social phobia. Eur Arch Psychiatry Clin Neurosci (suppl 1) 249:S11–S18, 1999

Bengel D, Greenberg BD, Cora-Locatelli G, et al: Association of the serotonin transporter promoter regulatory region polymorphism and obsessive-compulsive disorder. Mol Psychiatry 4:463–466, 1999

Benkelfat C, Murphy DL, Zohar J, et al: Clomipramine in obsessive-compulsive disorder: further evidence for a serotonergic mechanism of action. Arch Gen Psychiatry 46:23–28, 1989

Benkelfat C, Nordahl TE, Semple WE, et al: Local cerebral glucose metabolic rates in obsessive-compulsive disorder: patients treated with clomipramine. Arch Gen Psychiatry 47:840–848, 1990

Bienvenu OJ, Samuels JF, Riddle MA, et al: The relationship of obsessive-compulsive disorder to possible spectrum disorders: results from a family study. Biol Psychiatry 48:287–293, 2000

Billet EA, Richter MA, King N, et al: Obsessive compulsive disorder, response to serotonin reuptake inhibitors and the serotonin transporter gene. Mol Psychiatry 2:403–406, 1997

Birbaumer N, Grodd W, Diedrich O, et al: fMRI reveals amygdala activation to human faces in social phobics. Neuroreport 9:1223–1226, 1998

Black DW, Noyes R, Goldstein RB, et al: A family study of obsessive-compulsive disorder. Arch Gen Psychiatry 49:362–368, 1992

Brambilla F, Bellodi L, Perna G, et al: Dopamine function in obsessive-compulsive disorder: growth hormone response to apomorphine stimulation. Biol Psychiatry 42:889–897, 1997

Breiter HC, Rauch SL, Kwong KK, et al: Functional magnetic resonance imaging of symptom provocation in obsessive-compulsive disorder. Arch Gen Psychiatry 53:595–606, 1996

Bremner JD, Randall P, Scott TM, et al: MRI-based measurement of hippocampal volume in patients with combat-related posttraumatic stress disorder. Am J Psychiatry 152:973–981, 1995

Bremner JD, Licinio J, Darnell A, et al: Elevated CSF corticotropin-releasing factor concentrations in posttraumatic stress disorder. Am J Psychiatry 154:624–629, 1997a

Bremner JD, Randall P, Vermetten E, et al: Magnetic resonance imaging-based measurement of hippocampal volume in posttraumatic stress disorder related to childhood physical and sexual abuse: a preliminary report. Biol Psychiatry 41:23–32, 1997b

Bremner JD, Narayan M, Staib LH, et al: Neural correlates of memories of childhood sexual abuse in women with and without posttraumatic stress disorder. Am J Psychiatry 156:1787–1795, 1999a

Bremner JD, Staib LH, Kaloupek D, et al: Neural correlates of exposure to traumatic pictures and sound in Vietnam combat veterans with and without posttraumatic stress disorder: a positron emission tomography study. Biol Psychiatry 45:806–816, 1999b

Bremner JD, Innis RB, White T, et al: SPECT [I-123] iomazenil measurement of the benzodiazepine receptor in panic disorder. Biol Psychiatry 47:96–106, 2000

Buchsbaum MS, Wu J, Jaier R, et al: Positron emission tomography assessment of effects of benzodiazepines on regional glucose metabolic rate in patients with anxiety disorder. Life Sci 40:2393–2400, 1987

Capstick N, Seldrup V: Obsessional states: a study in the relationship between abnormalities occurring at birth and subsequent development of obsessional symptoms. Acta Psychiatr Scand 56:427–439, 1977

Carey G, Gottesman II: Twin and family studies of anxiety, phobic, and obsessive disorders, in Anxiety: New Research and Changing Concepts. Edited by Klein DF, Rabkin J. New York, Raven Press, 1981, pp 117–136

Cavallini MC, Di-Bella D, Pasquale L, et al: 5HT2C CYS23/SER23 polymorphism is not associated with obsessive-compulsive disorder. Psychiatry Res 77:97–104, 1998

Charney DS, Heninger GR: Abnormal regulation of noradrenergic function in panic disorders: effects of clonidine in healthy subjects and patients with agoraphobia and panic disorder. Arch Gen Psychiatry 43:1042–1054, 1986

Charney DS, Heninger GR, Breier A: Noradrenergic function in panic anxiety: effects of yohimbine in healthy subjects and patients with agoraphobia and panic disorder. Arch Gen Psychiatry 41:751–763, 1984

Charney DS, Goodman WK, Price LH, et al: Serotonin function in obsessive-compulsive disorder: a comparison of the effects of tryptophan and m-chlorophenylpiperazine in patients and healthy subjects. Arch Gen Psychiatry 45:177–185, 1988

Christensen KJ, Kim SW, Dysken MW, et al: Neuropsychological performance in obsessive compulsive disorder. Biol Psychiatry 31:4–18, 1992

Ciesielski KT, Beech HR, Gordon PK: Some electrophysiological observations in obsessional states. Br J Psychiatry 138:479–484, 1981

Cohen ME, White ID: Life situation, emotions, and neurocirculatory asthenia. Association for Research in Nervous and Mental Disease Proceedings 29:832–869, 1950

Comings DE, Muhleman D, Gysin R: Dopamine D2 receptor (DRD2) gene and susceptibility to posttraumatic stress disorder: a study and replication. Biol Psychiatry 40:368–372, 1996

Cooper PJ, Eke M: Childhood shyness and maternal social phobia: a community study. Br J Psychiatry 174:439–443, 1999

Coplan JD, Lydiard RB: Brain circuits in panic disorder. Biol Psychiatry 44:1264–1276, 1998

Coplan JD, Pine D, Papp L, et al: Uncoupling of the noradrenergic-hypothalamic-pituitary-adrenal axis in panic disorder patients. Neuropsychopharmacol 13:65–73, 1995

Coplan JD, Papp LA, Pine D, et al: Clinical improvement with fluoxetine therapy and noradrenergic function in patients with panic disorder. Arch Gen Psychiatry 54:643–648, 1997

Coupland NJ, Bell C, Potokar J, et al: Flumazenil challenge in social phobia. Anxiety 111:27- 30, 2000

Crowe RR, Noyes R, Pauls DL, et al: A family study of panic disorder. Arch Gen Psychiatry 40:1065–1069, 1983

Crowe RR, Wang Z, Noyes R, et al: Candidate gene study of eight GABAA receptor subunits in panic disorder. Am J Psychiatry 154:1096–1100, 1997

Curtis GC, Abelson JL, Gold PW: Adrenocorticotropic hormone and cortisol responses to corticotropin-releasing hormone: changes in panic disorder and effects of alprazolam treatment. Biol Psychiatry 41:76–85, 1997

Davis LL, Clark DM, Kramer GL, et al: D-fenfluramine challenge in posttraumatic stress disorder. Biol Psychiatry 45:928–930, 1999

DeBellis MD, Casey BJ, Dahl RE, et al: A pilot study of amygdala volumes in pediatric generalized anxiety disorder. Biol Psychiatry 48:51–57, 2000

Deckert J, Catalano M, Heils A, et al: Functional promoter polymorphism of the human serotonin transporter: lack of association with panic disorder. Psychiatr Genet 7:45–47, 1997

Deckert J, Nothen MM, Franke P, et al: Systematic mutation screening and association study of the A1 and A2a adenosine receptor genes in panic disorder suggest a contribution of the A2a gene to the development of the disease. Mol Psychiatry 3:81–85, 1998

Deckert J, Catalano M, Syagailo YV, et al: Excess of high activity monoamine oxidase A gene promoter alleles in female patients with panic disorder. Hum Mol Genet 81:228–234, 1999

Dorrow R, Horowski R, Paschelke G, et al: Severe anxiety induced by FG-7142, a beta-carboline ligand for benzodiazepine receptors. Lancet 1:98–99, 1983

Elam M, Yoat TP, Svensson TH: Hypercapnia and hypoxia: chemoreceptor-mediated control of locus ceruleus neurons and splanchnic, sympathetic nerves. Brain Res 222:373–381, 1981

Emmanuel NP, Lydiard BR, Ballenger JC: Treatment of social phobia with bupropion. J Clin Psychopharmacol 1:276–277, 1991

Ferrarese C, Appollonio I, Frigo M,et al: Decreased density of benzodiazepine receptors in lymphocytes of anxious patients: reversal after chronic diazepam treatment. Acta Psychiatr Scand 82:169–173, 1990

Flament MF, Rapoport JL, Murphy DL, et al: Biochemical changes during clomipramine treatment of childhood obsessive-compulsive disorder. Arch Gen Psychiatry 44:219–225, 1987

Flor-Henry P: The obsessive-compulsive syndrome, in Cerebral Basis of Psychopathology. Edited by Flor-Henry P. Boston, MA, John Coright, 1983, pp 301–311

Fredrikson M, Wik G, Greitz T, et al: Regional cerebral blood flow during experimental phobic fear. Psychophysiology 30:126–130, 1993

Freud S: Inhibitions, symptoms and anxiety (1926), in The Standard Edition of the Complete Psychological Works of Sigmund Freud, Vol 20. Translated and edited by Strachey J. London, Hogarth Press, 1959, pp 75–175

Frisch A, Michaelovsky E, Poyurovsky M, et al: Association between obsessive-compulsive disorder and polymorphisms of genes encoding components of the serotonergic and dopaminergic pathways. Eur Neuropsychopharmacol 10:205–209, 2000

Fyer AJ, Mannuzza S, Gallops MS, et al: Familial transmission of simple phobias and fears: a preliminary report. Arch Gen Psychiatry 47:252–256, 1990

Galderisi S, Mucci A, Catapano F, et al: Neuropsychological slowness in obsessive-compulsive patients: is it confined to tests involving the fronto-subcortical systems? Br J Psychiatry 167:394–398, 1996

Gelernter J, Southwick S, Goodson S, et al: No association between D2 dopamine receptor (DRD2) "A" system alleles, or DRD2 haplotypes, and posttraumatic stress disorder. Biol Psychiatry 45:620–625, 1999

Germine M, Goddard AW, Woods SW, et al: Anger and anxiety responses to m-chlorophenylpiperazine in generalized anxiety disorder. Biol Psychiatry 32:457–461, 1992

Giedd JN, Rapoport JL, Garvey MA, et al: MRI assessment of children with obsessive-compulsive disorder or tics associated with streptococcal infection. Am J Psychiatry 157:281–283, 2000

Gilbert AR, Moore GJ, Keshavan MS, et al: Decrease in thalamic volumes of pediatric patients with obsessive-compulsive disorder who are taking paroxetine. Arch Gen Psychiatry 57:449–456, 2000

Goddard AW, Mason GF, Almai A, et al: Reductions in occipital cortex GABA levels in panic disorder detected with 1H-magnetic resonance spectroscopy. Arch Gen Psychiatry 58:556–561, 2001

Gold M, Pottash AC, Sweeney DR, et al: Opiate withdrawal using clonidine. JAMA 243:343–346, 1980

Goldstein RB, Wickramaratne PJ, Horwath E, et al: Familial aggregation and phenomenology of 'early'-onset (at or before age 20 years) panic disorder. Arch Gen Psychiatry 54:271–278, 1997

Goodman WK, McDougle CJ, Price LH, et al: Beyond the serotonin hypothesis: a role for dopamine in some forms of obsessive compulsive disorder? J Clin Psychiatry 51 (suppl 8):36–43, 1990

Gorman JM, Levy GF, Liebowitz MR, et al: Effect of acute beta-adrenergic blockade on lactate-induced panic. Arch Gen Psychiatry 40:1079–1082, 1983

Gorman JM, Askanazi J, Liebowitz MR, et al: Response to hyperventilation in a group of patients with panic disorder. Am J Psychiatry 141:857–861, 1984

Gorman JM, Fyer MR, Goetz R, et al: Ventilatory physiology of patients with panic disorder. Arch Gen Psychiatry 45:31–39, 1988

Gorman JM, Liebowitz MR, Fyer AJ, et al: A neuroanatomical hypothesis for panic disorder. Am J Psychiatry 146:148–161, 1989a

Gorman JM, Battista D, Goetz RR, et al: A comparison of sodium bicarbonate and sodium lactate infusion in the induction of panic attacks. Arch Gen Psychiatry 46:145–150, 1989b

Gorman JM, Kent JM, Sullivan GM, et al: Neuroanatomical hypothesis of panic disorder, revised. Am J Psychiatry 157:493–505, 2000

Grimshaw L: Obsessional disorder and neurological illness. J Neurol Neurosurg Psychiatry 27:229–231, 1964

Han L, Nielsen DA, Rosenthal NE, et al: No coding variant of the tryptophan hydroxylase gene detected in seasonal affective disorder, obsessive-compulsive disorder, anorexia nervosa, and alcoholism. Biol Psychiatry 45:615–619, 1999

Hansenne M, Pitchot W, Ansseau M: The clonidine test in posttraumatic stress disorder (letter). Am J Psychiatry 148:810–811, 1991

Hayward C, Killen JD, Draemer HC, et al: Linking self-reported childhood behavioral inhibition to adolescent social phobia. J Am Acad Child Adolesc Psychiatry 37:1308–1316, 1998

Hewlett WA, Vinogradov S, Martin K, et al: Fenfluramine stimulation of prolactin in obsessive-compulsive disorder. Psychiatry Res 42:81–92, 1992

Hollander E, Liebowitz MR, Gorman JM, et al: Cortisol and sodium lactate-induced panic. Arch Gen Psychiatry 46:135–140, 1989

Hollander E, Schiffman E, Cohen Br, et al: Signs of central nervous system dysfunction in obsessive-compulsive disorder. Arch Gen Psychiatry 47:27–32, 1990

Hollander E, DeCaria C, Gully R, et al: Effects of chronic fluoxetine treatment on behavioral and neuroendocrine responses to meta-chlorophenylpiperazine in obsessive-compulsive disorder. Psychiatry Res 36:1–17, 1991a

Hollander E, DeCaria C, Nitescu A, et al: Noradrenergic function in obsessive-compulsive disorder: behavioral and neuroendocrine responses to clonidine and comparison to healthy controls. Psychiatry Res 37:161–177, 1991b

Hollander E, DeCaria CM, Nitescu A, et al: Serotonergic function in obsessive-compulsive disorder: behavioral and neuroendocrine responses to oral m-chlorophenylpiperazine and fenfluramine in patients and healthy volunteers. Arch Gen Psychiatry 49:21–28, 1992

Hollander E, Kwon J, Weiller F, et al: Serotonergic function in social phobia: comparison to normal control and obsessive-compulsive disorder subjects. Psychiatry Res 79:213–217, 1998

Horesh N, Amir M, Kedem P, et al: Life events in childhood, adolescence and adulthood and the relationship to panic disorder. Acta Psychiatr Scand 96:373–378, 1997

Insel TR, Mueller EA, Alterman I, et al: Obsessive-compulsive disorder and serotonin: is there a connection? Biol Psychiatry 20:1174–1188, 1985

Ishiguro H, Arinami T, Yamada K, et al: An association study between a transcriptional polymorphism in the serotonin transporter gene and panic disorder in a Japanese population. Psychiatry Clin Neurosci 51:333–335, 1997

Johnson M, Lydiard R, Zealberg J, et al: Plasma and CSF HVA levels in panic patients with comorbid social phobia. Biol Psychiatry 36:425–427, 1994

Johnson MR, Marazziti D, Brawman MO, et al: Abnormal benzodiazepine receptor density associated with generalized social phobia. Biol Psychiatry 43:306–309, 1998

Kagan J, Reznick JS, Snidman N: The physiology and psychology of behavioral inhibition in children. Child Dev 58:1459–1473, 1987

Karayiorgou M, Altemus M, Galke BL, et al: Genotype determining low catechol-O-methyltransferase activity as a risk factor for obsessive-compulsive disorder. Proc Natl Acad Sci USA 94:4572–4575, 1997

Karayiorgou M, Sobin C, Bludell ML, et al: Family based association studies support a sexually dimorphic effect of COMT and MAOA on genetic susceptibility to obsessive-compulsive disorder. Biol Psychiatry 45:1178–1189, 1999

Kardiner A: Traumatic neurosis of war, in American Handbook of Psychiatry, Vol 1. Edited by Arieti S. New York, Basic Books, 1959, pp 245–257

Kelly DD: The role of endorphins in stress-induced analgesia. Ann N Y Acad Sci 398:260–271, 1982

Kendler KS, Neale MC, Kessler RC, et al: Generalized anxiety disorder in women: a population-based twin study. Arch Gen Psychiatry 49:267–272, 1992a

Kendler KS, Neale MC, Kessler RC, et al: The genetic epidemiology of phobias in women: the interrelationship of agoraphobia, social phobia, situational phobia, and simple phobia. Arch Gen Psychiatry 49:273–281, 1992b

Kendler KS, Neale MC, Kessler RC, et al: Panic disorder in women: a population-based twin study. Psychol Med 23:397–406, 1993

Kennedy JL, Bradwejn J, Koszycki D, et al: Investigation of cholecystokinin system genes in panic disorder. Mol Psychiatry 4:284–285, 1999

Kim SJ, Veenstra-VanderWeele J, Hanna GL, et al: Mutation screening of human 5HT(2B) receptor gene in early onset obsessive-compulsive disorder. Mol Cell Probes 14:47–52, 2000

Klein DF: False suffocation alarms, spontaneous panics, and related conditions: an integrative hypothesis. Arch Gen Psychiatry 50:306–317, 1993

Knesevich JW: Successful treatment of obsessive-compulsive disorder with clonidine hydrochloride. Am J Psychiatry 139:364–365, 1982

Knowles JA, Fyer AJ, Vieland VJ, et al: Results of a genome-wide genetic screen for panic disorder. Am J Med Genet 81(2):139–147, 1998

Kolb LC: A neuropsychological hypothesis explaining posttraumatic stress disorders. Am J Psychiatry 144:989–995, 1987

Kolb LC, Burris BC, Griffiths S: Propranolol and clonidine in treatment of the chronic post-traumatic stress disorders of war, in Post-Traumatic Stress Disorder: Psychological and Biological Sequelae. Edited by van der Kolk BA. Washington, DC, American Psychiatric Press, 1984, pp 97–105

Kosten TR, Mason JW, Giller EL, et al: Sustained urine norepinephrine and epinephrine elevation in PTSD. Psychoneuroendocrinology 12:13–20, 1987

Leckman JF, Goodman WK, North WG, et al: Elevated cerebrospinal fluid levels of oxytocin in obsessive-compulsive disorder: comparison with Tourette's syndrome and healthy controls. Arch Gen Psychiatry 51:782–792, 1994

Lesch KP, Hoh A, Disselkamp-Tietze J, et al: 5-Hydroxytryptamine1A receptor responsivity in obsessive-compulsive disorder: comparison of patients and controls. Arch Gen Psychiatry 48:540–547, 1991

Levin P, Lazrove S, van der Kolk B: What psychological testing and neuroimaging tell us about the treatment of posttraumatic stress disorder by eye movement desensitization and reprocessing. J Anxiety Disord 13:159–172, 1999

Liebowitz MR, Fyer AJ, Gorman JM, et al: Lactate provocation of panic attacks, I: clinical and behavioral findings. Arch Gen Psychiatry 41:764–770, 1984

Liebowitz MR, Gorman JM, Fyer AJ, et al: Lactate provocation of panic attacks, II: biochemical and physiological findings. Arch Gen Psychiatry 42:709–719, 1985

Lucey JV, Barry S, Webb MG, et al: The desipramine-induced hormone response and the dexamethasone suppression test in obsessive-compulsive disorder. Acta Psychiatr Scand 86:367–370, 1992

Maier SF, Seligman ME: Learned helplessness: theory and evidence. J Exp Psychol 105:3–46, 1976

Maier SF, Dovies S, Gran JW: Opiate antagonists and long-term analgesic reaction induced by inescapable shock in rats. J Comp Physiol Psychol 94:1172–1183, 1980

Malizia AL, Cunningham VJ, Bell CJ, et al: Decreased brain GABA(A)-benzodiazepine receptor binding in panic disorder: preliminary results from a quantitative PET study. Arch Gen Psychiatry 55:715–720, 1998

Mason ST, Fibiger HC: Anxiety: the locus ceruleus disconnection. Life Sci 25:2141–2147, 1979

Mason JW, Giller EL, Kosten TR, et al: Urinary free-cortisol levels in posttraumatic stress disorder patients. J Nerv Ment Dis 174:145–149, 1986

Mason JW, Giller EL, Kosten TR, et al: Elevation of urinary norepinephrine/cortisol ratio in posttraumatic stress disorder. J Nerv Ment Dis 176:498–502, 1988

Mathew RJ, Ho BT, Kralik P, et al: Catecholamines and monoamine oxidase activity in anxiety. Acta Psychiatr Scand 63:245–252, 1981

McBride PA, DeMeo MD, Sweeney JA, et al: Neuroendocrine and behavioral responses to challenge with the indirect serotonin agonist dl-fenfluramine in adults with obsessive-compulsive disorder. Biol Psychiatry 31:19–34, 1992

McDougle CJ, Goodman WK, Price LH, et al: Neuroleptic addition in fluvoxamine-refractory obsessive-compulsive disorder. Am J Psychiatry 147:652–654, 1990

McGuire PK, Bench CJ, Frith CD, et al: Functional anatomy of obsessive-compulsive phenomena. Br J Psychiatry 164:459–468, 1994

McKeon J, McGuffin P, Robincon P: Obsessive-compulsive neurosis following head injury: a report of four cases. Br J Psychiatry 144:90–192, 1984

McNally RJ, Kohlbeck PA: Reality monitoring in obsessive-compulsive disorder. Behav Res Ther 31:24–53, 1993

Mikkelson EJ, Deltor J, Cohen DJ: School avoidance and social phobia triggered by haloperidol in patients with Tourette's syndrome. Am J Psychiatry 138:1572–1576, 1981

Miller HE, Deakin JF, Anderson IM: Effect of acute tryptophan depletion on CO_2-induced anxiety in patients with panic disorder and normal volunteers. Br J Psychiatry 176:182–188, 2000

Mountz JM, Modll JG, Wilson MW, et al: Positron emission tomographic evaluation of cerebral blood flow during state anxiety in simple phobia. Arch Gen Psychiatry 46:501–504, 1989

Mundo E, Maina G, Uslenghi C: Multicentre, double-blind, comparison of fluvoxamine and clomipramine in the treatment of obsessive-compulsive disorder. Int Clin Psychopharmacol 15:69–76, 2000

Murphy TK, Goodman WK, Fudge MW, et al: B lymphocyte antigen D8/17: a peripheral marker for childhood-onset obsessive-compulsive disorder and Tourette's syndrome? Am J Psychiatry 154:402–407, 1997

Nee LE, Caine ED, Polinsky RJ, et al: Gilles de la Tourette syndrome: clinical and family study of 50 cases. Ann Neurol 7:41–49, 1982

Nelson EC, Grant JD, Bucholz KK, et al: Social phobia in a population-based female adolescent twin sample: co-morbidity and associated suicide-related symptoms. Psychol Med 30:797–804, 2000

Nestadt G, Samuels J, Riddle M, et al: A family study of obsessive-compulsive disorder. Arch Gen Psychiatry 57:358–363, 2000a

Nestadt G, Lan T, Samuels J, et al: Complex segregation analysis provides compelling evidence for a major gene underlying obsessive-compulsive disorder and for heterogeneity by sex. Am J Hum Genet 67:1611–1616, 2000b

Noyes R Jr, Clarkson C, Crow RR, et al: A family study of generalized anxiety disorder. Am J Psychiatry 144:1019–1024, 1987

Nutt DJ: Altered central a2-adrenoreceptor sensitivity in panic disorder. Arch Gen Psychiatry 46:165–169, 1989

Nutt DJ, Glue P, Lawson C, et al: Flumazenil provocation of panic attacks: evidence for altered benzodiazepine receptor sensitivity in panic disorder. Arch Gen Psychiatry 47:917–925, 1990

Ohara K, Suzuki Y, Ochiai M, et al: A variable-number-tandem-repeat of the serotonin transporter gene and anxiety disorders. Prog Neuropsychopharmacol Biol Psychiatry 23:55–65, 1999

Ohman A, Soares JF: Unconscious anxiety: phobic responses to masked stimuli. J Abnorm Psychol 103:232–240, 1994

Otto MW: Normal and abnormal information processing. A neuropsychological perspective on obsessive-compulsive disorder. Psychiatr Clin North Am 15:825–848, 1992

Pacella BL, Polatin P, Nagler SH: Clinical and EEG studies in obsessive-compulsive states. Am J Psychiatry 100:830–838, 1944

Papp LA, Klein DF, Gorman JM: Carbon dioxide hypersensitivity, hyperventilation and panic disorder. Am J Psychiatry 150:1149–1157, 1993

Pauls DL, Towbin KE, Leckman JF, et al: Gilles de la Tourette's and obsessive-compulsive disorder: evidence supporting a genetic relationship. Arch Gen Psychiatry 43:1180–1182, 1986

Pavlov IP: Conditional Reflexes: An Investigation of the Physiological Activity of the Cerebral Cortex (1927). Edited by Anrep GV. New York, Dover, 1960

Perani D, Colombo C, Bressi S, et al: [18F] FDG PET study in obsessive-compulsive disorder: a clinical/metabolic correlation study after treatment. Br J Psychiatry 166:244–250, 1995

Perna G, Bussi R, Allevi L, et al: Sensitivity to 35% carbon dioxide in patients with generalized anxiety disorder. J Clin Psychiatry 60:379–384, 1999

Peroutka SJ, Price SC, Wilhoit TL, et al: Comorbid migraine with aura, anxiety and depression is associated with dopamine D2 receptor (DRD2) NcoI alleles. Mol Med 4:14–21, 1998

Perry BD, Giller EL Jr, Southwick SM: Altered plasma alpha-2-adrenergic binding sites in posttraumatic stress disorder (letter). Am J Psychiatry 144:1511–1512, 1987

Pigott TA, Hill JL, L'Heureux, et al: A comparison of the behavioral effects of oral versus intravenous m-CPP administration in OCD patients and the effect of metergoline prior to i.v. m-CPP. Biol Psychiatry 33:3–14, 1993

Pitman RK, Orr SP, Forgue DF, et al: Psychophysiologic assessment of posttraumatic stress disorder imagery in Vietnam combat veterans. Arch Gen Psychiatry 44:970–975, 1987

Pitman RK, van der Kolk BA, Orr SP, et al: Naloxone-reversible analgesic response to combat-related stimuli in posttraumatic stress disorder: a pilot study. Arch Gen Psychiatry 47:541–544, 1990

Pitts FN, McClure JN: Lactate metabolism in anxiety neurosis. N Engl J Med 277:1329–1336, 1967

Potts NL, Davidson JR, Krishnan KR, et al: Magnetic resonance imaging in social phobia. Psychiatr Res 52:35–42, 1994

Rainey JM Jr, Pohl RB, Williams M, et al: A comparison of lactate and isoproterenol anxiety states. Psychopathology 17 (suppl 1):74–82, 1984

Rainey JM Jr, Aleem A, Ortiz A, et al: Laboratory procedure for the inducement of flashbacks. Am J Psychiatry 144:1317–1319, 1987

Rapoport JL, Elkins R, Langer DH, et al: Childhood obsessive-compulsive disorder. Am J Psychiatry 138:1545–1554, 1981

Rauch SL, Jenike MA, Alpert NM, et al: Regional cerebral blood flow measured during symptom provocation in obsessive-compulsive disorder using oxygen 15-labeled carbon dioxide and positron emission tomography. Arch Gen Psychiatry 51:62–70, 1994

Rauch SL, Savage CR, Alpert NM, et al: A positron emission tomographic study of simple phobic symptom provocation. Arch Gen Psychiatry 52:20–28, 1995

Rauch SL, van der Kolk BA, Fisler RE, et al: A symptom provocation study of posttraumatic stress disorder using positron emission tomography and script-driven imagery. Arch Gen Psychiatry 53:380–387, 1996

Rauch SL, Whalen PJ, Shin LM, et al: Exaggerated amygdala response to masked facial stimuli in posttraumatic stress disorder: a functional MRI study. Biol Psychiatry 47:769–776, 2000

Redmond DE Jr: New and old evidence for the involvement of a brain norepinephrine system in anxiety, in Phenomenology and Treatment of Anxiety. Edited by Fann WE, Karacan I, Pokorny AD, et al. New York, Spectrum, 1979, pp 153–203

Rocca P, Beoni AM, Eva C, et al: Peripheral benzodiazepine receptor messenger RNA is decreased in lymphocytes of generalized anxiety disorder patients. Biol Psychiatry 43:767–773, 1998

Rosenberg DR, Keshavan MS: A.E. Bennett Research Award: toward a neurodevelopmental model of obsessive-compulsive disorder. Biol Psychiatry 43:623–640, 1998

Rosenberg DR, Keshavan MS, O'Hearn KM, et al: Frontostriatal measurement in treatment-naïve children with obsessive-compulsive disorder. Arch Gen Psychiatry 54:824–830, 1997

Rosenberg DR, Benazon NR, Gilbert A, et al: Thalamic volume in pediatric obsessive-compulsive disorder patients before and after cognitive behavioral therapy. Biol Psychiatry 48:294–300, 2000a

Rosenberg DR, MacMaster FP, Keshavan MS, et al: Decrease incaudate glutamatergic concentrations in pediatric obsessive-compulsive disorder patients taking paroxetine. J Am Acad Child Adolesc Psychiatry 39:1096–1103, 2000b

Rowe DC, Stever C, Gard JM, et al: The relation of the dopamine transporter gene (DAT1) to symptoms of internalizing disorders in children. Behav Genet 28:215–225, 1998

Roy-Byrne PP, Cowley DS, Greenblatt DJ, et al: Reduced benzodiazepine sensitivity in panic disorder. Arch Gen Psychiatry 47:534–538, 1990

Rubenstein CS, Peynircioglu ZF, Chambless DL, et al: Memory in sub-clinical obsessive-compulsive checkers. Behav Res Ther 31:759–765, 1993

Saletu ZG, Saletu B, Anderer P, et al: Nonorganic insomnia in generalized anxiety disorder. 1. Controlled studies on sleep, awakening and daytime vigilance utilizing polysomnography and EEG mapping. Neuropsychobiology 36:117–129, 1997

Schilder P: The organic background of obsessions and compulsions. Am J Psychiatry 94:1397-1416, 1938

Schindler KM, Richter MA, Kennedy JL, et al: Association between homozygosity at the COMT gene locus and obsessive-compulsive disorder. Am J Med Genet 96:721–724, 2000

Schneier F, Weiss U, Kessler C, et al: Subcortical correlates of differential classical conditioning of aversive emotional reactions in social phobia. Biol Psychiatry 45:863–871, 1999

Schneier F, Liebowitz MR, Abi-Dargham A, et al: Low dopamine D2 binding potential in social phobia. Am J Psychiatry 157:457–459, 2000

Schwartz JM, Stoessel PW, Baxter LR, et al: Systematic changes in cerebral glucose metabolic rate after successful behavior modification treatment in obsessive-compulsive disorder. Arch Gen Psychiatry 53:109–113, 1996

Schwartz C, Snidman N, Kagan J: Adolescent social anxiety as an outcome of inhibited temperament in childhood. J Am Acad Child Adolesc Psychiatry 38:1008–1015, 1999

Sevy S, Papadimitriou GN, Surmont DW, et al: Noradrenergic function in generalized anxiety disorder, major depressive disorder, and healthy subjects. Biol Psychiatry 25(2):141–152, 1989

Shin LM, Kosslyn SM, McNally RJ, et al: Visual imagery and perception in posttraumatic stress disorder: a positron emission tomographic investigation. Arch Gen Psychiatry 54:233–241, 1997

Skolnick P, Paul SM: Benzodiazepine receptors in the central nervous system. Int Rev Neurobiol 23:103–140, 1982

Skre I, Onstad S, Torgensen S, et al: A twin study of DSM-III-R anxiety disorders. Acta Psychiatr Scand 88:85–92, 1993

Smith MA, Davidson J, Ritchie JL, et al: The corticotropin releasing hormone test in patients with posttraumatic stress disorder. Biol Psychiatry 26:349–355, 1989

Southwick SM, Krystal JH, Morgan CA, et al: Abnormal noradrenergic function in posttraumatic stress disorder. Arch Gen Psychiatry 50:266–274, 1993

Southwick SM, Krystal JH, Bremner JD, et al: Noradrenergic and serotonergic function in posttraumatic stress disorder. Arch Gen Psychiatry 54:749–758, 1997

Spivak B, Vered Y, Graff E, et al: Low platelet-poor plasma concentrations of serotonin in patients with combat-related posttraumatic stress disorder. Biol Psychiatry 45:840–845, 1999

Stein MB, Asmundson GJ: Autonomic function in panic disorder: cardio-respiratory and plasma catecholamine responsivity to multiple challenges of the autonomic nervous system. Biol Psychiatry 36:548–558, 1994

Stein MB, Leslie WD: A brain single photon emission computed tomography (SPECT) study of generalized social phobia. Biol Psychiatry 39:825–828, 1996

Stein MB, Asmundson GJ, Chartier M: Autonomic responsivity in generalized social phobia. J Affect Disord 31:211–221, 1994

Stein MB, Millar TW, Larsen DK, et al: Irregular breathing during sleep in patients with panic disorder. Am J Psychiatry 152:1168–1173, 1995a

Stein MB, Delaney SM, Chartier M, et al: 3H paroxetine binding to platelets of patients with social phobia: comparison to patients with panic disorder and healthy volunteers. Biol Psychiatry 37:224–228, 1995b

Stein MB, Walker JR, Anderson G, et al: Childhood physical and sexual abuse in patients with anxiety disorders and in a community sample. Am J Psychiatry 153:275–277, 1996

Stein MB, Chartier MJ, Hazen AL, et al: A direct-interview family study of generalized social phobia. Am J Psychiatry 155:90–97, 1998a

Stein MB, Chartier MJ, Kozak MV, et al: Genetic linkage to the serotonin transporter protein and 5HT2A receptor genes excluded in generalized social phobia. Psychiatry Res 81:283–291, 1998b

Strohle A, Kellner M, Holsboer F, et al: Behavioral, neuroendocrine, and cardiovascular response to flumazenil: no evidence for an altered benzodiazepine receptor sensitivity in panic disorder. Biol Psychiatry 45:321–326, 1999

Swedo SE: Rituals and releasers: an ethological model of obsessive-compulsive disorder, in Obsessive-Compulsive Disorder in Children and Adolescents. Edited by Rapoport JL. Washington, DC, American Psychiatric Press, 1989, pp 269–288

Swedo SE, Rapoport JL, Cheslow DL, et al: Increased incidence of obsessive-compulsive symptoms in patients with Sydenham's chorea. Am J Psychiatry 146:246–249, 1989a

Swedo SE, Schapiro MB, Grady CL, et al: Cerebral glucose metabolism in childhood-onset obsessive-compulsive disorder. Arch Gen Psychiatry 46:518–523, 1989b

Swedo SE, Leonard HL, Kruesi MJP, et al: Cerebrospinal fluid neurochemistry in children and adolescents with obsessive-compulsive disorder. Arch Gen Psychiatry 49:29–36, 1992

Szeszko PR, Robinson D, Alvir JM, et al: Orbital frontal and amygdala volume reductions in obsessive-compulsive disorder. Arch Gen Psychiatry 56:913–919, 1999

Tancer ME, Stein MB, Uhde TW: Growth hormone response to intravenous clonidine in social phobia: comparison to patients with panic disorder and healthy volunteers. Biol Psychiatry 34:591–595, 1993

Tancer ME, Mailman RB, Stein MB, et al: Neuroendocrine responsivity to monoaminergic system probes in generalized social phobia. Anxiety 1:216–223, 1994

Thorén P, Åsberg M, Bertilsson L, et al: Clomipramine treatment of obsessive-compulsive disorder, II: biochemical aspects. Arch Gen Psychiatry 37:1289–1294, 1980

Tiihonen J, Kuikka J, Rasanen P, et al: Cerebral benzodiazepine receptor binding and distribution in generalized anxiety: a fractal analysis. Mol Psychiatry 2:463–471, 1997

Torgersen S: Genetic factors in anxiety disorders. Arch Gen Psychiatry 40:1085–1089, 1983

Towey J, Bruder G, Hollander E, et al: Endogenous event-related potentials in obsessive-compulsive disorder. Biol Psychiatry 28:92–98, 1990

True WR, Rice J, Eisen SA, et al: A twin study of genetic and environmental contributions to liability for posttraumatic stress symptoms. Arch Gen Psychiatry 50:257–264, 1993

Tweed JL, Schoenbach VJ, George LK, et al: The effects of childhood parental death and divorce on six-month history of anxiety disorders. Br J Psychiatry 154:823–828, 1989

Uhde TW, Tancer ME, Gelernter CS, et al: Normal urinary free cortisol and postdexamethasone cortisol in social phobia: comparison to normal volunteers. J Affect Disord 30:155–161, 1994

Van Den Hout M, Tenney N, Huygens K, et al: Preconscious processing bias in specific phobia. Behav Res Ther 35:29–34, 1997

van der Kolk BA, Saporta J: The biological response to psychic trauma: mechanisms and treatment of intrusion and numbing. Anxiety Research 4:199–212, 1991

van der Kolk BA, van der Hart O: Pierre Janet and the breakdown of adaptation in psychological trauma. Am J Psychiatry 146:1530–1540, 1989

van der Kolk BA, Boyd H, Krystal J, et al: Post-traumatic stress disorder as a biologically based disorder: implications of the animal model of inescapable shock, in Post-Traumatic Stress Disorder: Psychological and Biological Sequelae. Edited by van der Kolk BA. Washington, DC, American Psychiatric Press, 1984, pp 123–134

Van Der Linden G, van-Heerden B, Warwick J, et al: Functional brain imaging and pharmacotherapy in social phobia: single photon emission computed tomography before and after treatment with the selective serotonin reuptake inhibitor citalopram. Prog Neuropsychopharmacol Biol Psychiatry 24:419–438, 2000

Verburg C, Griez C, Meijer J: A 35% carbon dioxide challenge in simple phobias. Acta Psychiatr Scand 90:420–423, 1994

Wang Z, Valdes J, Noyes R, et al: Possible association of a cholecystokinin promoter polymorphism (CCK-36CT) with panic disorder. Am J Med Genet 81:228–234, 1998

Wilkinson DJ, Thompson JM, Lambert GW, et al: Sympathetic activity in patients with panic disorder at rest, under laboratory mental stress, and during panic attacks. Arch Gen Psychiatry 55:511–520, 1998

Wise SP, Rapoport JL: Obsessive-compulsive disorder: is it a basal ganglia dysfunction? in Obsessive-Compulsive Disorder in Children and Adolescents. Edited by Rapoport JL. Washington, DC, American Psychiatric Press, 1989, pp 327–344

Wu JC, Buchsbaum MS, Hershey TG, et al: PET in generalized anxiety disorder. Biol Psychiatry 29:1181–1199, 1991

Yehuda R, Southwick SM, Krystal JH, et al: Enhanced suppression of cortisol following dexamethasone administration in posttraumatic stress disorder. Am J Psychiatry 150:83–86, 1993

Yehuda R, Boisoneau D, Lowy MT, et al: Dose-response changes in plasma cortisol and lymphocyte glucocorticoid receptors following dexamethasone administration in combat veterans with and without posttraumatic stress disorder. Arch Gen Psychiatry 52:583–593, 1995

Zohar J, Mueller EA, Insel TR, et al: Serotonergic responsivity in obsessive-compulsive disorder: comparison of patients and healthy controls. Arch Gen Psychiatry 44:946–951, 1987

Zohar J, Insel TR, Zohar-Kadouch RC, et al: Serotonergic responsivity in obsessive-compulsive disorder: effects of chronic clomipramine treatment. Arch Gen Psychiatry 45:167–172, 1988

5

PSYCHOLOGICAL THEORIES

Despite the recent blossoming of biological psychiatry and our ever-increasing appreciation for the biological underpinnings of anxiety disorders, cognitive, behavioral, and psychodynamic perspectives remain invaluable in working with anxiety disorder patients. They help us think about the unique presentation of each individual, including what conflicts, cognitive biases, behavioral reinforcements, past adversities, and current stressors may be contributing to the onset or the exacerbation of symptoms. Psychological frameworks are also invaluable in informing and guiding our psychodynamic and cognitive-behavioral treatment approaches to the treatment of anxiety, many of which are highly effective.

■ PANIC DISORDER AND GENERALIZED ANXIETY DISORDER

Psychodynamic Theories

In his earliest concept of anxiety formation, Freud (1895a[1894]/1962) postulated that anxiety stems from the direct physiological transformation of libidinal energy into the somatic symptoms of anxiety, without the mediation of psychic mechanisms. He found evidence for this process in the sexual practices and experiences of patients with anxiety, which were characterized by disturbed sexual arousal and continence and coitus interruptus. He termed this kind of anxiety an *actual neurosis* as opposed to a *psychoneurosis*, because of the postulated absence of psychic processes. This anxiety, originating from overwhelming instinctual urges, would today be referred to as *id* or impulse anxiety. Over the next several years, Freud started to modify his theory. Although the basic tenet that anxiety stemmed from undischarged sexual energy remained the same, this was no longer posited to be due to external constraints such as sexual dysfunctions. In accordance with Freud's developing topographic theory of the mind, anxiety resulted from forbidden sexual drives in the unconscious being repressed by the preconscious.

By 1926, with the advent of the structural theory of the mind, Freud's theory of anxiety had undergone a major transformation (Freud 1926/1959). Anxiety was now an affect belonging to the ego and acted as a "signal," alerting the ego to internal danger. The danger stems from intrapsychic conflict between instinctual drives from the id, prohibitions from the superego, and the demands of external reality. Anxiety acts as a signal to the ego for the mobilization of repression and other defenses to counteract the threat to intrapsychic equilibrium. Inhibitions and neurotic symptoms develop as measures designed to avoid the dangerous situation and to allow only partial gratification of instinctual wishes, thus warding off signal anxiety. In the revised theory, then, anxiety leads to repression, instead of the reverse.

Early in his work, Freud (1895b[1894]/1962) also observed that in the analysis of phobias, anxiety played a prominent role. He stated that in the case of agoraphobia we often find the recollection of an anxiety attack, and what the patient actually fears is the occurrence of such an attack under the special conditions in which he believes he cannot escape it. This is a succinct description, more than a century ago, of the development of anticipatory anxiety and agoraphobia following a panic attack. At that time, Freud did not consider phobias to be psychologically mediated. Rather, he understood them, like anxiety neurosis, to be manifestations of a physiologically induced tension state. Undischarged libidinal energy was physiologically transformed into anxiety, which became attached to and partly discharged through objects that were, by their nature or in the patient's prior experience, dangerous.

The intrapsychic conflict model of anxiety continues to constitute a major tenet of contemporary psychoanalytic theory. Psychoanalytic theorists after Freud, such as Melanie Klein (1948) and Joachim Flescher (1955), also made major contributions to the understanding of the psychodynamic origins of anxiety. Whereas Freud concentrated on the role of sexual impulses and the oedipal conflict in the genesis of anxiety, these theorists drew attention to the role that aggressive impulses and preoedipal dynamics can also play in generating anxiety. In the time since Freud, the psychodynamic literature has also, to a degree, shifted away from formulations that primarily emphasize libidinal wishes and castration fears to other ways of understanding phobias such as agoraphobia (Michels et al. 1985). For example, the significance of a trustworthy and safe companion to a person with agoraphobia could be understood as a simultaneous expression of aggressive impulses toward the companion and a magical wish to protect the companion from those impulses by always being together. Alternatively, excessive fear of object loss and its concomitant separation anxiety could explain both the fear of being away from home alone and the alleviation of this fear when a companion is present.

Although psychoanalytic theories of panic are not universally accepted today, they remain an invaluable tool in the understanding and treatment of at least some patients. Also, it should be pointed out that Freud's theory of anxiety formation is not incompatible with biological theories of anxiety. Although Freud's first model of anxiety was later overshadowed by the conflictual model, modern biological theories of panic are in many ways more reminiscent of his original physiological formulation. Furthermore, Freud maintained on numerous occasions that biological predispositions to psychiatric symptoms are undoubtedly operant in most conditions and that constitutional factors could play a role in the particular form that neurotic symptoms take in different patients. What psychoanalytic theory does not help us with is a better understanding of the determinants of the various specific forms in which anxiety manifests itself. Some patients have panic attacks; others have more chronic forms of anxiety; and still others have phobias, obsessions, or compulsions. Freud himself had attempted to address this problem of choice of neurosis and partly explained it on the basis of constitutional factors—a concept essentially similar to modern biological notions.

In an attempt to reconcile the unpredictability in choice of symptoms with classical psychodynamic theory, theorists have postulated that patients with unconscious conflict and a neural predisposition to panic may perhaps manifest their anxiety in the form of panic attacks, whereas individuals without this neural predisposition may possibly manifest milder forms of signal anxiety (Nemiah 1981). Along these more contemporary lines of thinking, results of a psychodynamic study of patients with panic disorder suggested that in patients who are neurophysiologically predisposed to early-age fearfulness, exposure to parental behaviors that augment this fearfulness can result in disturbances of object relations, persistence of conflicts surrounding dependence, and catastrophic fears of helplessness that may all be accessible in psychodynamic treatment (Shear et al. 1993).

With the broadening of psychodynamic theory over the decades and increasing research in infant and child development, attachment theory and the potential importance of attachment disturbances in the genesis of psychopathology have become an area of great interest. In the early 1960s, D. F. Klein advanced an etiologic theory that agoraphobia with panic attacks may represent an aberrant function of the biological substrate that underlies normal human attachment and threats to it—that is, separation anxiety. On the basis of work by Bowlby (1973) on attachment and separation, Klein (1981) advanced the notion that the attachment of an infant animal or human to its mother is not simply a learned response, but is genetically programmed and biologically determined. Indeed, 20%–50% of adults with panic disorder and agoraphobia recall manifesting symptoms of pathological separation anxiety—often taking the form of school phobia—when they were children. Furthermore, the initial panic attack in the history of a patient who goes on to develop panic disorder is sometimes preceded by the real or threatened loss of a important relationship. One systematic study showed that the number and severity of recent life events, especially events related to loss, were greater in new-onset panic disorder patients than in control subjects (Faravelli and Pallanti 1989). A psychodynamic study showed separation anxiety to be a much more prevalent theme in the dreams and screen memories of patients with panic than in healthy control subjects, as assessed by blinded raters (Free et al. 1993).

Infant animals demonstrate their protest anxiety, when separated from their mother, by a series of high-pitched cries, called *distress vocalizations*. Imipramine has been found to be effective in blocking distress vocalizations in dogs (Scott 1975) and in monkeys (Suomi et al. 1978). Imipramine is a highly effective antipanic drug in adult humans. Hypothesizing a link between adult panic attacks and childhood separation anxiety, Gittelman-Klein and Klein (1971) conducted a study of imipramine treatment for children with school phobia. In these children, fear of separation from their mothers was usually the basis behind refusing to go to school. The drug proved successful in getting the children to return to school. In a related finding, Weissman et al. (1984) found three times as much risk of separation anxiety in children who had parents with panic disorder as in children whose parents did not.

Thus, evidence suggests that the same drug that diminishes protest anxiety in higher mammals also reduces separation anxiety in children and blocks panic attacks in adults. This evidence provided further confirmation of the link between separation anxiety and panic attacks. Is early separation anxiety linked to agoraphobia or also to panic attacks? If imipramine affects panic attacks, and separation anxiety is linked to agoraphobia, then why is imipramine effective in the treatment of school phobia? On the other hand, children with school phobia do not have spontaneous panic attacks, but this distinction could be related to their young age. Perhaps both panic disorder and panic disorder with agoraphobia are linked to a biologically disordered separation mechanism that is responsive to imipramine. It is possible that the retrospective histories of a lesser degree of separation anxiety in patients with panic attacks alone are misremembered.

Contemporary psychoanalysts, in response, have claimed that this neurophysiological and ethological model of a disrupted separation mechanism and panic disorder may be unnecessarily reductionistic (Michels et al. 1985). They point out an inconsistency between the conceptualization of panic attacks as spontaneous and the frequently reported histories of childhood separation anxiety in patients with panic attacks, and state that psychological difficulties with separation can also play a role in subsequent vulnerability to panic attack. On the other hand, contemporary psychoanalysts have also given more credence to the role of biological substrates in the genesis of anxiety symptoms in at least some patients who have developed their anxious personality structure secondary to a largely contentless biologic dysregulation, so that although psychological triggers for anxiety may still be found, the anxiety threshold is so low in these patients that it is no longer useful to view the psychological event as etiologically significant (Cooper 1985).

Behavioral Theories

Behavioral theorists hold that anxiety is conditioned by the fear of certain environmental stimuli. If every time a laboratory animal presses a bar it receives a noxious electric shock, the pressing of the lever becomes a *conditioned stimulus* that precedes the *unconditioned stimulus* (i.e., the shock). The conditioned stimulus releases a *conditioned response* in the animal (anxiety) that leads the animal to avoid contact with the lever, thereby avoiding the shock. Successful avoidance of the unconditioned stimulus, the shock, reinforces the avoidant behavior. This avoidance leads to a decrease in anxiety level. By analogy with this animal model, we might say that anxiety attacks are conditioned responses to fearful situations. For example, an infant learns that if his or her mother is not present (i.e., the conditioned stimulus) he or she will experience hunger (i.e., the unconditioned stimulus), and the infant learns to become anxious automatically whenever the mother is absent (i.e., the conditioned response). The anxiety may persist even after the child is old enough to feed himself or herself. To give another example, a life-threatening situation in someone's life (e.g., skidding in a car during a snowstorm) is paired with the experience of rapid heartbeat (i.e., the conditioned stimulus) and tremendous anxiety. Long after the accident, rapid heartbeat alone, whether during vigorous exercise or minor emotional upset, becomes capable by itself of provoking the conditioned response of an anxiety attack.

Certain problems are posed by such a theory. First, although some traumatic situations—a symptomatic episode in thyroid disease, cocaine intoxication, or a life-threatening event such as a suffocation incident—do seem to be paired with the onset of panic disorder, for many patients no such traumatic event can ever be pinpointed. An interesting note: traumatic suffocation incidents have been found in about 20% of panic disorder patients, markedly more than in psychiatric comparison subjects (Bouwer and Stein 1997). Clinical experience also does not support the idea that anxiety disorder patients undergo repeated traumatic events and therefore should be able to extinguish their anxiety. So even though learning theories have a powerful basis in experimental animal research, they do not seem to explain adequately, on their own, the pathogenesis of human anxiety disorders. However, coupled with a dysregulated biological mechanism or vulnerability that may be linked to the process of fear conditioning in panic disorder—such as altered functioning of the amygdala and related fear circuits (see Chapter 4, "Biological Theories")—heightened anxiety responses could conceivably persist over time.

Cognitive Theories

There is evidence for specificity in cognitive content in the various anxiety disorders. For example, panic disorder patients have more cognitions related to physical catastrophes (Breitholtz et al. 1999), whereas patients with generalized anxiety disorder (GAD) demonstrate more cognitions in the categories of interpersonal confrontation, competence, acceptance, concern about others, and worry over minor matters. Specific types of information-processing biases also appear to facilitate the cognitions characteristic of panic disorder and GAD. Compared to control subjects, persons with panic disorder demonstrate an attentional bias towards threatening rather than positive words (McNally et al. 1997). In addition, a bias for physical-threat words in explicit, but not implicit, memory processes has been demonstrated in persons with panic disorder relative to subjects without a psychiatric disorder (Lundh et al. 1997). Similarly in GAD, a bias for threat-related information in implicit memory processes has been described (MacLeod and McLaughlin 1995); selective attentional biases for threatening information (Mogg et al. 1999, Mogg et al. 2000); and difficulty with decision making when faced with ambiguity (MacLeod and Cohen 1993).

Cognitive distortions characteristic of panic disorder involve two major components. One is the interpretation of the uncomfortable physical sensations associated with panic attacks as dangerous or catastrophic—for example, that one is about to faint, die, or have a heart attack. The other component is the irrational thoughts of catastrophe regarding the situational consequences of having panic attacks—for example, the beliefs that one will be ridiculed, humiliated, or in danger of losing a job or a relationship.

In terms of the etiology of GAD, cognitive theory speculates a relationship to early cognitive schemata (Table 5–1), born from negative experiences of the world as a dangerous place (Barlow 1988) or insecure and anxious early attachments to important caregivers (Cassidy 1995). Distinct cognitive processes underlying the origins versus the maintenance of GAD have been eloquently summarized in recent work (Aikins and Craske 2001). Regarding the origins of GAD, it has been proposed that insecure attachment relationships, ambivalence toward caregivers, as well as parental overprotection and lack of emotional warmth, may all contribute to later development of GAD. Additional mechanisms contribute to perpetuating GAD. First, worry is used as a strategy for avoiding intense negative affects. Second, worry about unlikely and future threat removes the need to deal with more proximal and realistic threats and limits the capacity to find solutions to more immediate conflicts. Finally, individuals with GAD engage in a certain degree of magical thinking and believe that their worry helps prevent a feared outcome, thus

TABLE 5–1.	Cognitive schemata characteristic of generalized anxiety disorder

History of insecure attachments and ambivalence toward parental figures[a]

History of parental overprotection and lack of emotional warmth

View of the world as a dangerous place[b]

Fear of interpersonal confrontations

Doubts regarding self-competence and acceptability[c]

Use of worry to avoid intense negative affects[c]

Worrying about future unlikely threats, as a distraction from more proximal realistic fears[c]

Magical thinking that worrying about a bad outcome will somehow prevent its happening[c]

[a]Cassidy 1995. [b]Barlow 1988. [c]Aikins and Craske 2001.

leading to a negative reinforcement of the process of worrying (Aikins and Craske 2001). There is also evidence that the process of meta-worry (i.e., worrying about worrying) contributes to the high degree of pathological worry in GAD (Wells and Carter 1999).

■ SOCIAL PHOBIA

Psychodynamic Theories

In the classic psychodynamic formulation of phobias they are viewed as compromise formations used to deal with forbidden and anxiety-provoking sexual or aggressive wishes, often of an oedipal nature, leading to the mobilization of three defensive steps: projection, displacement, and avoidance—and thus development of a phobia. In this framework, then, one way of conceptualizing performance anxiety is as a fear of audiences compensating for an underlying wish to excel, succeed, and be admired, with all their associated imagined dangers.

From an object relations theory and a more pre-oedipal perspective, social phobia may be understood as a consequence of early internalized object relations characterized by socially-damaging important others who are critical, harsh, ridiculing, or humiliating.

These harsh introjects from childhood are then projected in later years onto other persons in one's life, resulting in social anxiety (Gabbard 1992). Alternatively, children with socially fearful or inept parents may from an early age internalize powerful ego-building identifications with those figures, leading to later problems with social anxiety.

Behavioral Theories

A number of behavioral mechanisms have been proposed that may contribute to the pathogenesis of social phobia (Table 5–2). These include direct exposure to socially related traumatic events; vicarious learning through observing others engaged in those traumatic situations; and information transfer—that is, the things one hears in various contexts regarding social interactions (Ost 1987; Stemberger et al. 1995). There is a notable familial component to social phobia, part of which is thought to be heritable and part acquired. Parents, whether socially anxious themselves or not, might rear socially anxious children through various mechanisms such as not providing exposure to social situations and development of social skills, overprotectiveness, controlling and critical behavior, modeling of socially anxious behaviors, and conveying fearful information about social situations (Hudson and Rapee 2000). For example, in an experimental paradigm it has been shown that socially ambiguous situations are interpreted favorably by children without socially phobic parents but avoidantly when family input is negative (Dadds et al. 1996).

Cognitive Theories

A number of cognitive distortions can be identified in persons with established social phobia, all centering on various manifestations of a core negative representation of one's social self (Table 5–2). There is evidence that persons with social phobia do not habituate to negative social information as easily as nonanxious control subjects (Amir et al. 2001). They also exhibit an implicit memory bias

TABLE 5–2.	Behavioral and cognitive mechanisms in social phobia
Behavioral[a]	Direct exposure to socially related traumatic events
	Vicarious learning through observing and modeling after others with socially anxious behaviors
	Information transfer, negative information from various contexts regarding social interactions
	Lack of adequate exposure to social situations and development of social skills
	Parental overprotectiveness
	Parental controlling and critical behavior
Cognitive[b]	Core negative representation of one's social self
	Greater cognitive flexibility in interpreting anxiety symptoms exhibited by others, but more judgmental about one's own anxiety symptoms
	Negative interpretations of ambiguous social events
	Catastrophic interpretations of mildly negative social events
	Negative expectation that social success will result in greater future social demands

[a]Data from Hudson and Rapee 2000; Ost 1987; Stemberger et al. 1995.
[b]Data from Amir et al. 1998a; Roth et al. 2001; Stopa and Clark 2000; Wallace and Alden 1997.

for socially threatening information (Amir et al. 2000), more flexibility in interpreting anxiety symptoms exhibited by others but a more judgmental interpretation of their own (Amir et al. 1998a, Roth et al. 2001), negative interpretations of ambiguous social events and catastrophic interpretations of mildly negative social events (Stopa and Clark 2000), and a negative expectation that social success will result in greater future social demands (Wallace and Alden 1997). Children with social phobia, compared to their nonaxious peers, have been found to have social skills deficits, more negative self-talk, less competent social performance with peers, and fewer positive outcomes from peers (Spence et al. 1999). In an information-processing paradigm, persons with social phobia were found to exhibit higher vigilance and avoidance of threatening information than control subjects (Amir et al. 1998b).

■ SPECIFIC PHOBIAS

Psychodynamic Theories

As stated previously, in the classic psychodynamic formulation of phobias they are viewed as compromise formations resulting from the projection, displacement, and avoidance of forbidden and anxiety-provoking sexual or aggressive wishes. In Freud's well-known case history of Little Hans, these processes were first eloquently elaborated (Freud 1909/1955). Little Hans was a 5-year-old boy who developed a phobia of horses. Through an analysis of the boy's conversations with his parents, Freud hypothesized that as a compromise to the anxiety aroused by his sexual feelings for his mother and the guilty fear of retribution and castration from his father, Little Hans projected and displaced his anxiety onto a "safe" third object, horses. He thus could avoid the ambivalence inherent in his original conflict, because he both hated and also loved his father, and could regulate his anxiety by avoiding horses, but at the cost of becoming housebound. Individual exploration for possible psychodynamic components to specific phobia remains useful, although it is probably fair to say that cognitive-behavioral models have now become more prevalent in understanding this form of psychopathology.

Behavioral Theories

In learning theory, specific phobia is thought to be a conditioned response acquired through association of the phobic object (i.e., the conditioned stimulus) with a noxious experience (the unconditioned stimulus). (In this chapter, in the first section, "Panic Disorder and Generalized Anxiety Disorder," see the subsection "Behavioral Theories.") Initially, the noxious experience (e.g., an electric shock) produces an unconditioned response of pain, discomfort, and fear. If a person frequently receives an electric shock when in contact with the phobic object, then by contiguous conditioning the appearance of the phobic object alone may come to elicit an anxiety response (i.e., conditioned response). Avoidance of the phobic object prevents or reduces this conditioned anxiety and is therefore perpetuated through drive reduction. This classical learning theory model of phobias has received much reinforcement from the relative success of behavioral (i.e., *deconditioning*) techniques in the treatment of many patients with specific phobias. However, the model has also been criticized on the grounds that it is not consistent with a number of empirically observed aspects of phobic behavior in humans.

Models regarding the etiology of specific phobias have been recently elaborated and critiqued by Fyer (1998). She describes that in order to satisfactorily explain specific phobia, a *modified conditioning model* would be needed, on four counts. First, many patients with specific phobia do not recall an initial aversive event, suggesting that if such an event had occurred it must be encoded by amygdala-based emotional memory but not by hippocampal-based episodic memory, either because it occurred before age 3 or because it was encoded under highly stressful conditions. Second, it turns out that a very small number of objects account for most of human phobias, suggesting that there may be an evolutionarily wired biological preparedness toward specific stimuli that would be easily conditioned but difficult to extinguish. Third, only a minority of persons exposed to a particular stimulus develop a phobic reaction—suggesting that additional factors such as genetic vulnerabilities or previous experiences play a role. Fourth, most specific phobias are resistant to extinction in the absence of specific interventions, despite belief and evidence that there is nothing to fear.

Another model of specific phobias is the *nonassociative learning model* (Fyer 1998), which is in a sense the converse of the conditioned model above. It proposes that each species has certain innate fears that are part of normal development and that essentially what goes wrong in specific phobia is a failure to habituate over time to these intrinsic developmental fears. This nonhabituation could be due to various processes such as stressful life events, constitutional vulnerabilities, or unsafe environments.

■ OBSESSIVE-COMPULSIVE DISORDER

Psychodynamic Theories

Before 1980 and the advent of DSM-III (American Psychiatric Association 1980), obsessive-compulsive disorder (OCD) was classified as obsessive-compulsive neurosis, a psychodynamically conceptualized neurotic state, a concept that now is probably more useful in understanding the dynamics of obsessive-compulsive personality disorder. Obsessional neurosis was seen as the outcome of a regression from oedipal conflicts to the earlier anal psychosexual stage, facilitated by possibly preexisting anal fixations. The typical defenses associated with obsessionalism include isolation of affect and intellectualization, reaction formation, and doing-undoing. Obsessional doubt and indecision, which at its worse can be extremely time-consuming or even paralyzing, can be understood in terms of the heightened ambivalence and difficulty integrating the good with the bad that results from the anal regression. In some cases, it was also believed that an obsessional veneer helped protect at least some more primitive patients who had a psychotic core from more serious psychotic decompensation.

Behavioral Theories

A prominent behavioral model for the acquisition and maintenance of obsessive-compulsive symptoms derives from the two-stage learning theory of Mowrer (1939). In stage 1, anxiety is classically conditioned to a specific environmental event (i.e., classical conditioning). The person then engages in compulsive rituals (escape or avoidance responses) in order to decrease anxiety. If the person is successful in reducing anxiety, the compulsive behavior is more likely to occur in the future (stage 2, operant conditioning). Higher-order conditioning occurs when other neutral stimuli such as words, images, or thoughts are associated with the initial stimulus and the associated anxiety is diffused. Ritualized behavior preserves the fear response, because the person avoids the eliciting stimulus and thus avoids extinction. Likewise, anxiety reduction following the ritual preserves the compulsive behavior.

Cognitive Theories

Certain types of cognitions and cognitive processes are highly characteristic of OCD, and presumably contribute, if not to the genesis, then at least to the maintenance of the disorder. In particular, negative beliefs about responsibility, especially responsibility surrounding intrusive cognitions, may be a key factor influencing obsessive behavior (Salkovskis et al. 2000). Study participants with OCD also appeared to have memory biases toward disturbing themes—for example, better memory for contaminated objects—than control subjects with comparable memory (Radomsky and Rachman 1999). Persons with OCD who check have been found not to have memory impairments, which presumably could account for the excessive checking, but rather low confidence in their memory (MacDonald et al. 1997). Persons with OCD have also been found to have deficits in selective attention, and it has been proposed that those deficits may relate to their diminished ability to selectively ignore intrusive cognitive stimuli (Clayton et al. 1999). Deficits in spatial working memory, spatial recognition, and motor initiation and execution have also been found in OCD (Purcell et al. 1998). In contrast to adults, neuropsychological deficits have not been found in children in OCD, suggesting that OCD symptoms may not interfere with cognition earlier in the illness (Beers et al. 1999).

■ POSTTRAUMATIC STRESS DISORDER

Psychodynamic Theories

Traditional psychodynamic theory, dating back to Freud's rejection of the seduction model in favor of intrapsychic fantasies and conflicts, is widely viewed as having had a rather destructive impact on the study of trauma until the past 20 years, when various astute researchers and clinicians such as Mardi Horowitz (1976) and Judith Herman (1997) began to elaborate the psychodynamics of trauma. Posttraumatic stress disorder (PTSD) cannot be reconciled with one's preexisting schemata of the self and its relationship to the world. It therefore can result in widespread affective dysregulation, trouble tolerating impulses and conflicts that were previously better contained, and activation of more primitive and repressed object relations. A number of themes can potentially be activated after trauma, including overwhelming loss and grief; guilt over surviving; feelings of helplessness, hopelessness, lack of safety, and meaninglessness about the future; frightening and guilt-ridden wishes for revenge and empowerment; feelings of shame and guilt. The identification of the basic themes that may be most active in any given person, and the way in which these are related to pre-existing conflicts and further hamper recovery from trauma, can be very useful. One very important idea to bring away from classic psychodynamic theory is that no matter how horrendous a given trauma, humans are creatures of mind and meaning and will unavoidably elaborate any traumatic experience with personal and idiosyncratic meanings. One common scenario is the traumatic consequences of rape, which so often include not only the typical symptoms of PTSD, but feelings of guilt and shame that have little to do with the external reality of what occurred and that can be fruitfully explored psychodynamically.

Behavioral Theories

Behavioral theory suggests that there is a disturbance of conditioned responses in PTSD. Autonomic responses to both innocuous and aversive stimuli are elevated, with greater responses to unpaired cues and reduced extinction of conditioned responses (Peri et al. 2000). It is proposed that persons with PTSD have higher arousal of the sympathetic system at the time of conditioning and therefore are more conditionable than trauma-exposed persons without PTSD (Orr et al. 2000). Persons with PTSD also generalize fear-related conditioned responses from a variety of stimuli, having been sensitized by stress (Grillon and Morgan 1999).

Cognitive Theories

A cognitive model has been proposed for the persistence of PTSD symptoms, suggesting that PTSD becomes persistent when persons process trauma in ways that lead to an ongoing sense of serious and current threat. This processing occurs by excessively negative appraisals of the trauma or its consequences, and by a disturbance of autobiographical memory so that there is poor contextualization and strong associative memory (Ehlers and Clark 2000).

Recent studies have revealed a number of disturbances in cognitive processes associated with PTSD. For example, the high incidence of PTSD after severe traumatic brain injury with loss of consciousness and few traumatic memories suggests that trauma can mediate PTSD in part at an implicit level (Bryant et al. 2000). Impairments in explicit memory have been associated with PTSD (Bremner et al. 1993, Jenkins et al. 1998) and may be related to hippocampal toxicity resulting from stress-mediated elevations in cortisol (Bremner et al. 1995). In addition, persons who have PTSD may not exhibit recall deficits for trauma-related words, but rather for positive and neutral words—suggesting that avoiding the encoding of disturbing information does not occur in PTSD (McNally et al. 1998). This characteristic appears consistent with the intrusive nature of traumatic memories clinically encountered in the disorder. Indeed, there appears to be an attentional bias towards traumatic stimuli in PTSD (Bryant and Harvey 1997), whereas generalized attentional disturbances have not been found (Golier et al. 1997).

■ REFERENCES

Aikins DE, Craske MG: Cognitive theories of generalized anxiety disorder. Psychiatr Clin North Am 24:57–74, 2001

American Psychiatric Association: Diagnostic and Statistical Manual of Mental Disorders, 3rd Edition. Washington, DC, American Psychiatric Association, 1980

Amir N, Foa EB, Coles ME: Negative interpretation bias in social phobia. Behav Res Ther 36:945–957, 1998a

Amir N, Foa EB, Coles ME: Automatic activation and strategic avoidance of threat-relevant information in social phobia. J Abnorm Psychol 107:285–290, 1998b

Amir N, Foa EB, Coles ME: Implicit memory bias for threat-relevant information in individuals with generalized social phobia. J Abnorm Psychol 109:713–720, 2000

Amir N, Coles ME, Brigidi B, et al: The effect of practice on recall of emotional information in individuals with generalized social phobia. J Abnorm Psychol 110:76–82, 2001

Barlow DH: Anxiety and Its Disorders: The Nature and Treatment of Anxiety and Panic. New York, Guilford, 1988

Beers SR, Rosenberg DR, Dick EL, et al: Neuropsychological study of frontal lobe function in psychotropic-naïve children with obsessive-compulsive disorder. Am J Psychiatry 156:777–779, 1999

Bouwer C, Stein DJ: Association of panic disorder with a history of traumatic suffocation. Am J Psychiatry 154:1566–1570, 1997

Bowlby J: Attachment and Loss, Vol 2: Separation: Anxiety and Anger. New York, Basic Books, 1973

Breitholtz E, Johansson B, Ost LG: Cognitions in generalized anxiety disorder and panic disorder patients: a prospective approach. Behav Res Ther 37:533–544, 1999

Bremner JD, Scott TM, Delaney RC, et al: Deficits in short-term memory in posttraumatic stress disorder. Am J Psychiatry 150:1015–1019, 1993

Bremner JD, Randall P, Scott TM, et al: MRI-based measurement of hippocampal volume in patients with combat-related posttraumatic stress disorder. Am J Psychiatry 152:973–981, 1995

Bryant RA, Harvey AG: Attentional bias in posttraumatic stress disorder. J Trauma Stress 10:635–644, 1997

Bryant RA, Marosszeky JE, Crooks J, et al: Posttraumatic stress disorder after severe traumatic brain injury. Am J Psychiatry 157:629–631, 2000

Cassidy J: Attachment and generalized anxiety disorder, in Rochester Symposium on Developmental Psychopathology, Vol 6: Emotion, Cognition and Representation. Edited by Cicchetti D, Toth S. Rochester, NY, University of Rochester Press, 1995

Clayton IC, Richards JC, Edwards CJ: Selective attention in obsessive-compulsive disorder. J Abnorm Psychol 108:171–175, 1999

Cooper AM: Will neurobiology influence psychoanalysis? Am J Psychiatry 142:1395–1402, 1985

Dadds MR, Barrett PM, Rapee RM, et al: Family process and child anxiety and aggression: an observational analysis. J Abnorm Child Psychol 24:187–203, 1996

Ehlers A, Clark DM: A cognitive model of posttraumatic stress disorder. Behav Res Ther 38:319–345, 2000

Faravelli C, Pallanti S: Recent life events and panic disorder. Am J Psychiatry 146:622–626, 1989

Flescher J: A dualistic viewpoint on anxiety. J Am Psychoanal Assoc 3:415–446, 1955

Free NK, Winget CN, Whitman RM: Separation anxiety in panic disorder. Am J Psychiatry 150:595–599, 1993

Freud S: Analysis of a phobia in a five-year-old boy (1909), in The Standard Edition of the Complete Psychological Works of Sigmund Freud, Vol 10. Translated and edited by Strachey J. London, Hogarth Press, 1955, pp 1–149

Freud S: Inhibitions, symptoms and anxiety (1926), in The Standard Edition of the Complete Psychological Works of Sigmund Freud, Vol 20. Translated and edited by Strachey J. London, Hogarth Press, 1959, pp 75–175

Freud S: On the grounds for detaching a particular syndrome from neurasthenia under the description anxiety neurosis (1895a[1894]), in The Standard Edition of the Complete Psychological Works of Sigmund Freud, Vol 3. Translated and edited by Strachey J. London, Hogarth Press, 1962, pp 85–117

Freud S: Obsessions and phobias (1895b[1894]), in The Standard Edition of the Complete Psychological Works of Sigmund Freud, Vol 3. Translated and edited by Strachey J. London, Hogarth Press, 1962, pp 69–84

Fyer AJ: Current approaches to etiology and pathophysiology of specific phobia. Biol Psychiatry 44:1295–1304, 1998

Gabbard GO: Psychodynamics of panic disorder and social phobia. Bull Menninger Clin 52:A3-A13, 1992

Gittelman-Klein R, Klein DF: Controlled imipramine treatment of school phobia. Arch Gen Psychiatry 25:204–207, 1971

Golier J, Yehuda R, Cornblatt B, et al: Sustained attention in combat-related posttraumatic stress disorder. Integr Physiol Behav Sci 32:52–61, 1997

Grillon C, Morgan CA: Fear-potentiated startle conditioning to explicit and contextual cues in Gulf War veterans with posttraumatic stress disorder. J Abnorm Psychol 108:134–142, 1999

Herman J: Trauma and Recovery. Basic Books, New York, NY, 1997

Horowitz MJ: Stress-response syndromes: a review of posttraumatic and adjustment disorders. Hosp Community Psychiatry 37:241–249, 1976

Hudson J, Rapee R: The origins of social phobia. Behav Modif 24:102–129, 2000

Jenkins MA, Langlasi PJ, Delis D, et al: Learning and memory in rape victims with posttraumatic stress disorder. Am J Psychiatry 155:278–279, 1998

Klein DF: Anxiety reconceptualized, in Anxiety: New Research and Changing Concepts. Edited by Klein DF, Rabkin JG. New York, Raven, 1981, pp 235–263

Klein M: A contribution to the theory of anxiety and guilt. Int J Psychoanal 29:114–123, 1948

Lundh LG, Czyzykow S, Ost LG: Explicit and implicit memory bias in panic disorder with agoraphobia. Behav Res Ther 35:1003–1014, 1997

MacDonald PA, Antony MM, Macleod CM, et al: Memory and confidence in memory judgments among individuals with obsessive compulsive disorder and non-clinical controls. Behav Res Ther 35:497–505, 1997

MacLeod C, Cohen IL: Anxiety and the interpretation of ambiguity: a text comprehension study. J Abnorm Psychol 2:102, 1993

MacLeod C, McLaughlin K: Implicit and explicit memory bias in anxiety: a conceptual replication. Behav Res Ther 33:1–14, 1995

McNally RJ, Hornig CD, Otto MW, et al: Selective encoding of threat in panic disorder: application of a dual priming paradigm. Behav Res Ther 35:543–549, 1997

McNally RJ, Metzger LJ, Lasko NB, et al: Directed forgetting of trauma cues in adult survivors of childhood sexual abuse with and without posttraumatic stress disorder. J Abnorm Psychol 107:596–601, 1998

Michels R, Frances A, Shear MK: Psychodynamic models of anxiety, in Anxiety and the Anxiety Disorders. Edited by Tuma AH, Maser JD. Hillsdale, NJ, Erlbaum, 1985, pp 595–618

Mogg K, Mathews A, Weinman J: Selective processing of threat cues in anxiety states: a replication. Behav Res Ther 27:317–323, 1999

Mogg K, Millar N, Bradley BP: Biases in eye movements to threatening facial expressions in generalized anxiety disorder and depressive disorder. J Abnorm Psychol 109:695–704, 2000

Mowrer O: A stimulus response analysis of anxiety and its role as a reinforcing agent. Psychol Rev 46:553–565, 1939

Nemiah JC: A psychoanalytic view of phobias. Am J Psychoanal 41:115–120, 1981

Orr SP, Metzger LJ, Lasko NB, et al: De novo conditioning in trauma-exposed individuals with and without posttraumatic stress disorder. J Abnorm Psychol 109:290–298, 2000

Ost LG: Age of onset of different phobias. J Abnorm Psychol 96:223–229, 1987

Peri T, Ben Shakhar G, Orr SP, et al: Psychophysiologic assessment of aversive conditioning in posttraumatic stress disorder. Biol Psychiatry 47:512–519, 2000

Purcell R, Maruff P, Kyrios M, et al: Neuropsychological deficits in obsessive-compulsive disorder: a comparison with unipolar depression, panic disorder, and normal controls. Arch Gen Psychiatry 55:415–423, 1998

Radomsky AS, Rachman S: Memory bias in obsessive-compulsive disorder (OCD). Behav Res Ther 37:605–618, 1999

Roth D, Antony MM, Swinson RP: Interpretations for anxiety symptoms in social phobia. Behav Res Ther 39:129–138, 2001

Salkovskis PM, Wroe AL, Gledhill A, et al: Responsibility attitudes and interpretations are characteristic of obsessive compulsive disorder. Behav Res Ther 38:347–372, 2000

Scott JP: Effects of psychotropic drugs on separation distress in dogs, in Proceedings of the IX Congress of Neuropsychopharmacology, Amsterdam, Excerpta Medica, 1975, pp 735–745

Shear MK, Cooper AM, Klerman GL, et al: A psychodynamic model of panic disorder. Am J Psychiatry 150:859–866, 1993

Spence SH, Donovan C, Brechman, et al: Social skills, social outcomes, and cognitive features of childhood social phobia. J Abnorm Psychol 108:211–221, 1999

Stemberger RT, Turner SM, Beidel DC, et al: Social phobia: an analysis of possible developmental factors. J Abnorm Psychol 104:526–531, 1995

Stopa L, Clark DM: Social phobia and interpretation of social events. Behav Res Ther 38:273–283, 2000

Suomi SJ, Seaman SF, Lewis JK, et al: Effects of imipramine treatment of separation-induced social disorders in rhesus monkeys. Arch Gen Psychiatry 35:321–325, 1978

Wallace ST, Alden LE: Social phobia and positive social events: the price of success. J Abnorm Psychol 106:416–424, 1997

Weissman MM, Leckman JF, Merikangas KR, et al: Depression and anxiety disorders in parents and children: results from the Yale family study. Arch Gen Psychiatry 41:845–852, 1984

Wells A, Carter K: Preliminary tests of a cognitive model of generalized anxiety disorder. Behav Res Ther 37:585–594, 1999

6

SOMATIC TREATMENTS

■ PANIC DISORDER

The central goal in the treatment of panic disorder is the pharmacological blockade of the panic attacks. Several classes of medication have been shown to be effective in accomplishing this aim, and a summary of the pharmacological treatment of panic disorder is presented in Table 6–1. When a drug regimen is initiated for a patient with panic disorder, it is crucial for the patient to understand that the drug will block the panic attacks but may not necessarily decrease the amount of intervening anticipatory anxiety and avoidance, at least initially. For patients with severe anxiety, it can be helpful to initially prescribe a concomitant benzodiazepine, which can be gradually tapered and discontinued after several weeks of antidepressant treatment (Goddard et al. 2001). Also important, some patients with panic disorder display an initial hypersensitivity to antidepressants, whether tricyclic antidepressants (TCAs) or serotonin reuptake inhibitors, and complain of jitteriness, agitation, a feeling of speed, and insomnia. Although this hypersensitivity is usually transient, it is one of the main reasons why panic patients may opt early to discontinue medication. Therefore, it is strongly recommended that patients with panic disorder be given lower doses of antidepressants initially than would be given to depressed patients.

Tricyclic Antidepressants

The most widely studied medications in the past were the TCAs, especially imipramine (Klein 1964; Mavissakalian and Michelson

TABLE 6–1.   **Pharmacological treatment of panic disorder**

Selective serotonin reuptake inhibitors

General indications: First-line, alone or in combination with benzodiazepines if needed; also first choice with comorbid OCD, GAD, depression, and social phobia; start at very low doses and increase; response seen with low to moderate doses

Specific medications

   Sertraline, paroxetine: FDA approved

   Fluvoxamine, fluoxetine, citalopram: appear similarly efficacious

Tricyclic antidepressants

General indications: Established efficacy, second line if SSRIs fail or not tolerated

Specific medications

   Imipramine: well studied

   Clomipramine: high efficacy but not easily tolerated

   Desipramine: if patient has low tolerance to anticholinergic side effects

   Nortriptyline: if patient is prone to orthostatic hypotension, elderly

Monoamine oxidase inhibitors

General indications: Poor response to or poor tolerance of other antidepressants; comorbid atypical depression or social phobia without good SSRI response

Specific medications

   Phenelzine: most studied MAOI

   Tranylcypromine: less sedation than phenelzine

High-potency benzodiazepines

General indications: Poor response to or tolerance of antidepressants; prominent anticipatory anxiety or phobic avoidance; initial treatment phase until antidepressant begins to work

Specific medications

   Clonazepam: longer-acting, less frequent dosing, less withdrawal, first choice

   Alprazolam: well studied but short-acting

Other medications

Other antidepressants: *Venlafaxine* and *nefazodone*: less studied but seem efficacious

TABLE 6–1. **Pharmacological treatment of panic disorder** *(continued)*

Other options: Particularly as augmentation for patients whose
conditions are refractory or for those who are intolerant of all above
medications; not well tested to date:
  Pindolol: effective augmentation in one controlled trial
  Valproic acid: open trials only
  Inositol: open trials only
  Clonidine: in open trials, initial response that later tends to fade

Note. "FDA approved" refers to approval specifically for use in the disorder
named in the table title. Comparisons made in any section on specific medications refer to medications in that section only, unless otherwise stated. FDA =
U.S. Food and Drug Administration; GAD = generalized anxiety disorder; OCD
= obsessive-compulsive disorder; SSRI = selective serotonin reuptake inhibitor.

1986a, 1986b; McNair and Kahn 1981; Sheehan et al. 1980; Zitrin
et al. 1980; Zitrin et al. 1983). Other TCAs, such as desipramine,
are also effective, although they have not been studied as extensively as imipramine. Nortriptyline has not been systematically
studied, but clinical experience indicates it also is efficacious. The
presence of depressed mood is not a predictor or requirement in order for these drugs to be effective in blocking panic attacks. In recent years, the selective serotonin reuptake inhibitors (SSRIs) have
been shown to be efficacious in treating panic disorder, and, given
their several advantages over TCAs, they have become the first-line
treatment for panic disorder. TCAs are now reserved, for the most
part, for patients who do not have a good response to, or do not tolerate, selective serotonin reuptake inhibitors and related medications.

A standard TCA regimen is for the patient to start with imipramine 10 mg at bedtime and increase the dose by 10 mg every
other night until 50 mg is reached (po). The dosage can be taken all
at once. Because 50 mg is usually inadequate for full panic blockade, the dosage can then be raised by 25-mg increments every
3 days, or by 50-mg increments weekly, to a maximum of 300 mg/
day. Most patients need at least 150 mg/day of TCA, and, unfortu-

nately, underdosage commonly occurs. In some cases, a dosage of imipramine greater than 300 mg is necessary. With imipramine dosing of about 200 mg/day, more than 80% of patients show a marked reduction in the number of panic attacks (Mavissakalian and Perel 1989). Panic disorder patients for whom "high" doses of imipramine are not effective should have blood TCA levels measured. Often, blood levels will be disproportionately low for the dosage, suggesting rapid metabolism or excretion, malabsorption, or noncompliance on the part of the patient. It appears that patients do not show further antipanic responses at combined plasma levels beyond 140 mg/mL (Mavissakalian and Perel 1995). Patients who experience excessive anticholinergic side effects to imipramine can take desipramine instead. Elderly patients or patients who are otherwise very sensitive to orthostatic hypotension can try nortriptyline.

Serotonin Reuptake Inhibitors

A number of open and controlled treatment trials have now documented that the potent serotonin reuptake blockers are highly effective in the treatment of panic disorder. Given their higher safety and ease of administration compared with TCAs, they have become the first-line treatment in panic disorder, either alone or in combination with benzodiazepines when needed. As a first-line treatment, they also offer the advantage of being effective for several commonly comorbid disorders, such as depression, social phobia, generalized anxiety disorder (GAD), and obsessive-compulsive disorder (OCD). Although only paroxetine and sertraline are approved by the U.S. Food and Drug Administration (FDA) for panic disorder, there is no particular reason to think that all SSRIs do not have comparable efficacy in panic disorder. Several controlled trials have documented the efficacy of fluvoxamine in dosages up to 150 mg/day (Den Boer 1988; Hoehn-Saric et al. 1993). The efficacy of paroxetine has also been demonstrated in controlled trials, at dosages of 20–60 mg/day, according to one study (Oehrberg et al. 1995). In another study, however, only the 40-mg/day dosage reached statistically significant superiority over placebo during a 10-week period, whereas the 10-mg and 20-mg doses did not, thus highlighting the importance of trying higher doses if response to lower doses is inadequate (Ballenger et al. 2000). Not surprisingly, another paroxetine study documented that it was as efficacious as clomipramine in treating panic disorder but better tolerated (Lecrubier et al. 1997). Both medications retained their efficacy during a continued blinded-study maintenance period of 9 months, leading to further patient improvement and highlighting the importance of longer-term treatment (Lecrubier and Judge 1997). In large controlled trials, the SSRI sertraline has also been found to be efficacious in treating panic disorder (Londborg et al. 1998; Pohl et al. 1998). Sertraline not only markedly decreased the number of panic attacks, but also led to significant improvement in patients' quality of life and had a low dropout rate (Pohl et al. 1998). In contrast to the paroxetine study, no difference was shown among three sertraline dosages—50 mg, 100 mg, or 200 mg/day—in reducing panic attacks (Londborg et al. 1998). It is interesting to note that a prior history of benzodiazepine use does not affect the tolerability or response to sertraline treatment, regardless of whether the response to the benzodiazepine had been good or bad (Rapaport et al. 2001). Still another SSRI, citalopram, has been shown to be efficacious in treating panic disorder. In an acute 8-week controlled trial, the middle dosage of 20–30 mg/day conferred the most advantageous benefit-risk ratio compared with the higher and lower dosages used (Wade et al. 1997). In a 1-year controlled maintenance extension of the prior study, the lowest dosage of 10–15 mg/day was not better than placebo, whereas the middle dosage of 20–30 mg/day again showed the best response (Lepola et al. 1998). Fluoxetine is similarly efficacious in treating panic disorder. Fluoxetine, especially at a dosage of 20 mg/day, rather than 10 mg/day, has been shown to be superior to placebo in the acute treatment of panic disorder (Michelson et al. 1998). Interestingly, the study that reported these findings used a wide range of measures and demonstrated that broad improvement was more related to phobia, anxiety, depression, and impairment than to panic attacks per se, again highlighting the importance of looking at the larger picture when assessing change.

During a 6-month maintenance treatment period, the randomized controlled study continued; participants for whom acute fluoxetine treatment was initially effective demonstrated further major improvement if they were placed in the study group that received fluoxetine and significant worsening if placed in the group that received placebo (Michelson et al. 1999). Clomipramine has been used in dosages of 25–200 mg/day, titrated to patients' individual responses, and appears at least as efficacious and better tolerated at lower doses compared with higher doses in treating panic attacks and, to a lesser degree, avoidance (Caillard et al. 1999). However, it is generally less well tolerated than SSRIs in panic disorder (Lecrubier et al. 1997) and therefore is generally not a first-line treatment.

One meta-analytic study found that serotonin reuptake inhibitors emerged superior to imipramine and to alprazolam in treating panic, but lower doses of the latter two may have partly accounted for this difference (Boyer 1995). Like the TCAs, SSRIs can cause uncomfortable overstimulation in panic patients if started at the usual doses. It is therefore strongly recommended that treatment be started gingerly at 5–10 mg/day for fluoxetine, 10 mg/day for paroxetine and citalopram, and 25 mg/day (or even 12.5 mg/day) for sertraline and fluvoxamine. The dose can then be gradually increased to an average dose by weekly adjustments. A moderate or lower daily dose is usually adequate for most patients, as described in the reports of the trials mentioned earlier, and high doses are generally not needed and less well tolerated.

Monoamine Oxidase Inhibitors

Monoamine oxidase inhibitors (MAOIs) are as effective as the TCAs and the SSRIs in treating panic. Both phenelzine and tranylcypromine successfully treat panic disorder; phenelzine has been studied more extensively. Phenelzine can be started at 15 mg/day, taken in the morning. The dosage is then increased by 15 mg every 4–7 days as tolerated, up to a maximum of 60–90 mg/day. If sedation or weight gain is of concern, tranylcypromine may be tried, starting at 10 mg in the morning, and increasing by 10 mg every 4 days to a maximum of 80 mg/day. Serotonin reuptake inhibitors and TCAs are typically preferred over MAOIs because they are better tolerated and they obviate the need for dietary restrictions and the risk of hypertensive crises. Furthermore, patients who do not respond to a TCA or a serotonin reuptake inhibitor alone may respond to a combination of the two (Tiffon et al. 1994). However, MAOIs are an option to consider for patients who are not able to tolerate or to respond well to other antidepressants. In patients with concomitant atypical depression or social phobia, MAOIs may be an appropriate earlier choice for treatment if SSRIs do not confer adequate results.

Benzodiazepines

Although clinicians prefer to use antidepressants for the first-line treatment of panic disorder, high-potency benzodiazepines are also highly effective in treating the condition. In one study, 82% of patients treated acutely with alprazolam showed at least moderate improvement in panic disorder, compared with 43% who were taking placebo. Onset of response was rapid, with notable improvement occurring in the first weeks of treatment, and the mean final dosage was 5.7 mg/day. After 8 weeks of acute treatment, patients were withdrawn from medication, with dosages tapered over a period of 4 weeks; 27% of the patients experienced rebound panic attacks and 35% had withdrawal symptoms. After discontinuation, panic disorder outcome for the alprazolam-treated group was not significantly different from that for the placebo group (Pecknold et al. 1988). Clonazepam appears equally promising in the acute treatment of panic disorder, according to a large, multicenter trial (Rosenbaum et al. 1997). In the acute treatment of panic attacks, the lowest dosage of 0.5 mg/day was least efficacious; dosages of 1 mg/day or higher (2 mg, 3 mg, and 4 mg/day) were equally efficacious, and the dosages of 1–2 mg/day were better tolerated. Long-term efficacy, possible tolerance and dependency, and difficulties in discontinuing the medication are the main areas of concern when choosing benzodiazepine treatment. Results of naturalistic follow-up studies of long-term benzodiazepine treatment appear generally optimistic, because most patients maintain their therapeutic gains without increasing their benzodiazepine dose over time (Nagy et al. 1989; Schweizer et al. 1993).

These medications have fewer initial side effects than TCAs and serotonin reuptake inhibitors. However, the general treatment principle is that anxiolytics should be reserved until the different classes of antidepressants have failed, because they do pose some risk of tolerance, dependence, and withdrawal problems. For patients with severe acute distress and disability, who require immediate relief, the indication might be to start treatment with a benzodiazepine and then replace it with an antidepressant. There is also some evidence that benzodiazepines may be more effective, at least initially, in ameliorating the associated anticipatory anxiety and phobic avoidance—another possible indication for their initial use. Systematic comparisons of antidepressants and benzodiazepines in the acute and maintenance treatment of panic disorder have shown that patients treated with alprazolam are significantly more likely to stay in treatment and experience relief from their panic attacks than patients taking imipramine; the latter is associated with worse patient compliance (Schweizer et al. 1993).

Clonazepam should generally be preferred as a first choice, because it is longer acting and thus has the advantages of less frequent dosing (twice or even once a day) and less risk of withdrawal symptoms than alprazolam. Clonazepam should generally be started at 0.5 mg bid, and increased only if needed, usually to a maximum dosage of 4 mg/day. Alprazolam is usually started at 0.5 mg qid and is gradually increased to an average dosage of 4 mg/day, in a range of 2–10 mg/day according to the individual patient. Treatment for at least 6 months is recommended, as with the antidepressants. Patients' moods while taking these drugs must be followed, because alprazolam may occasionally cause mania, and clonazepam can cause depression. Discontinuation must be gradual to prevent withdrawal symptoms; a reduction of 15% of the total dose weekly is generally a safe regimen, but an even slower rate may be required to prevent the recurrence of panic. In a controlled study one-third of patients were unable to tolerate a 4-week tapering of alprazolam after 8 months of maintenance treatment; the strongest predictor of taper failure was the initial severity of panic attacks rather than the alprazolam dose (Rickels et al. 1993a). The distinction between actual withdrawal symptoms and a simple recrudescence of the original anxiety symptom, when the benzodiazepine is stopped, remains controversial, and this distinction can be difficult to make clinically. It has been convincingly shown that the introduction of cognitive-behavioral therapy greatly increases the likelihood that panic disorder patients will be able to successfully discontinue their benzodiazepine medication by tapering (Otto et al. 1993; Spiegel et al. 1994).

Although benzodiazepines are generally safe, with side effects limited mainly to sedation, there is a concern that some patients may become tolerant or even addicted to these medications. Available data indicate, however, that most patients are able to stop taking them without serious sequelae and that the problem of tolerance and dependence is overestimated and probably limited to an addiction-prone population, or to patients with refractory panic disorder who may escalate standard benzodiazepine use in attempts at self-medication. A recent study suggested that combining a benzodiazepine (clonazepam) with an SSRI (sertraline) on initiation of treatment leads to a rapid antipanic response, and then tapering the benzodiazepine after the SSRI takes effect could be accomplished without adverse effect (Goddard et al. 2001).

Other Medications

Venlafaxine, a combined serotonin-norepinephrine inhibitor (SNRI), led to the recession of panic attacks in four patients treated openly with low dosages of 50–75 mg/day (Geracioti 1995) and has been found to be efficacious in one controlled study (Pollack et al. 1996). It, therefore, definitely merits further study, and clinically it should be a consideration when SSRIs do not work well. Nefazodone, a serotonin reuptake inhibitor and serotonin type 2 (5-HT$_2$) antagonist, also appears promising in treating panic: in another study, 70% of 14 patients treated openly for 8 weeks with dosages of 200–600 mg/day notably improved (DeMartinis et al. 1996). Nefazodone was again shown to have some efficacy in treating panic disorder in another small open trial (Papp et al. 2000). If the results can be replicated in a larger controlled study, this medication may hold some benefits, in terms of initial anxiogenic response and long-term sexual side effects, compared with SSRIs.

Buspirone, a serotonin (5-HT$_{1A}$) agonist nonbenzodiazepine antianxiety agent, has not been found effective in treating panic. Similarly, there is no evidence that beta-adrenergic blocking drugs, such as propranolol, are effective in blocking spontaneous panic attacks. If panic attacks occur in a specific social context, such as public speaking, a trial of beta-blocker would be indicated.

Clonidine, which inhibits locus coeruleus discharge, would seem for theoretical reasons to be a good antipanic drug. Although in a small-series study two-thirds of patients responded initially, the therapeutic effect tends to be lost in a matter of weeks despite continuation of dose (Liebowitz et al. 1981). A later study confirmed a similar pattern of loss of response during a 10-week trial (Uhde et al. 1989). This loss of response, plus a number of bothersome side effects, makes clonidine a poor initial choice for treatment of panic disorder. However, one controlled study found clonidine to be efficacious for both panic disorder and GAD (Hoehn-Saric et al. 1981).

When effectiveness of SSRIs and other antidepressants has been inadequate, one augmentation strategy, shown to be effective in a small, blinded trial, may be to add pindolol 2.5 mg tid (Hirschmann et al. 2000).

Valproic acid may also have some beneficial effects in the treatment of panic attacks (Keck et al. 1993). In one open trial, all of 12 patients were moderately to markedly improved after 6 weeks of treatment, and 11 continued the medication and maintained their gains after 6 months (Woodman and Noyes 1994). Controlled trials, however, have not been reported. A fairly large controlled trial of another mood stabilizer, gabapentin, at flexible dosages of 600–3600 mg/day, showed it to be no better than placebo in treating panic disorder (Pande et al. 2000), although a post hoc analysis showed it to have some efficacy in the more severely symptomatic patients, suggesting that an augmentation study in refractory panic disorder might be worthwhile

Inositol, an intracellular second messenger precursor, was found to be effective in treating panic disorder in a placebo-controlled 4-week trial at a dosage of 12 g/day (Benjamin et al. 1995), but this result has not been replicated.

Prognosis and Course of Treatment

Full remission of panic attacks with antidepressants usually requires 4–12 weeks of treatment. Subsequently, the duration of required treatment in order to prevent relapse is a function of the natural course of panic disorder. The disorder can probably best be characterized as chronic, with an exacerbating and remitting course. Therefore, complete agreement among researchers and clinicians has not been reached regarding the recommended course of treatment. In a naturalistic follow-up study, Noyes and his group found that the majority of panic disorder patients initially treated with TCAs had a relatively good prognosis—followed during a few years—whether they had stayed on medication (60% of the sample) or had stopped it (40% of the sample) (Noyes et al. 1989). In a somewhat less optimistic, but controlled and prospective study, a very high relapse rate for panic disorder was found when imipramine was discontinued after 6 months of acute treatment. However, half-dose imipramine—about 80 mg/day—was successful in preventing relapse during 1 year of maintenance treatment (Mavissakalian and Perel 1992). Thus, a reasonable recommendation for treating patients with panic disorder is to have them take full-dose medication for at least 6 months, after which time, medication can be tapered to half-dose, and patients should be followed to ensure that clinical improvement is maintained. Subsequently, the clinician may attempt gradual dose decreases every few months as long as the improvement is maintained, to reach a minimal dose on which the patient is relatively symptom-free. Some patients may eventually be able to completely discontinue medications, while others will not.

■ GENERALIZED ANXIETY DISORDER

The pharmacological treatment of GAD is summarized in Table 6–2. Although the major changes in the diagnostic criteria in consecutive editions of DSM, the presence of frequent comorbidity in GAD, and the tendency to view GAD as a secondary or minor condition had hampered past treatment research. Pharmacotherapy options have expanded in recent years and will probably continue to expand in the near future with the development of new classes of antianxiety medications.

Anxiolytics

In past years, benzodiazepines have been the first-line treatment of GAD, and they continue to be a first-line option today, despite certain concerns over their chronic use and newer first-line medication choices such as buspirone, SSRIs and SNRIs. A number of controlled studies clearly show that chronically anxious patients respond well to benzodiazepines, and all benzodiazepines are probably similarly efficacious in treating GAD (Rickels et al. 1983, Ruiz 1983). There is some evidence that benzodiazepines may be more effective in treating the physical symptoms of anxiety, while antidepressants, whether TCAs or SSRIs, may be more effective in treating the psychic symptoms (Hoehn-Saric et al. 1988; Rocca et al. 1997). It has also been suggested that benzodiazepines such as chlordiazepoxide may peak in effectiveness after 4 weeks of treatment, whereas TCAs such as imipramine may be more effective for patients with anxiety over the longer term (Kahn et al. 1986). Although benzodiazepines are generally safe, with side effects limited mainly to sedation and slowed mentation, there is a concern that some patients may become tolerant or even addicted to these medications. However, available data indicate that the concern over benzodiazepine abuse in chronically anxious populations is overestimated, and in reality most patients continue to derive clinical benefits without developing abuse or dependence (Romach et al. 1995). Concerns about addiction are probably jus-

TABLE 6–2.	Pharmacological treatment of generalized anxiety disorder

Venlafaxine extended-release

General indications: First-line treatment; FDA approved; proven efficacy in large controlled trials; generally well tolerated; once-a-day dosing; recommended starting dose is 75 mg/day, which may be adequate for a number of patients

Selective serotonin reuptake inhibitors

General indications: First-line treatment

Specific medications

Paroxetine: proven efficacy in large controlled trials; FDA approved; well tolerated; once-a-day dosing; recommended starting dose is 20 mg/day, which may be adequate for many patients

Other SSRIs: have not been extensively tested but are similarly efficacious

Benzodiazepines

General indications: Well-known efficacy and widely used; all appear similarly efficacious; patients may be monitored for dependence and withdrawal symptoms; benzodiazepines may be more effective for the physical rather than cognitive symptoms of GAD

Buspirone

General indications: Proven efficacy; well tolerated; a trial is generally indicated in all patients; compared with benzodiazepines, buspirone takes longer to take action and is not associated with a "high"; there may be less efficacy and compliance in patients recently treated with benzodiazepines

Tricyclic antidepressants

General indications: Shown efficacy in few trials; more side effects than benzodiazepines, buspirone, and newer antidepressants; delayed action compared with benzodiazepines; may be more effective for cognitive rather than physical symptoms of anxiety

Specific medications

Imipramine: shown efficacy

Trazodone: shown efficacy

160

TABLE 6–2. **Pharmacological treatment of generalized anxiety disorder** *(continued)*

Other medications

Nefazodone: one open trial

Mirtazapine: one open trial with comorbid major depression

Clonidine: tends to lose initial response

Propranolol: may be useful adjuvant in patients with pronounced palpitations and tremor

---

Note. "FDA approved" refers to approval specifically for use in the disorder named in the table title. Comparisons made in any section on specific medications refer to medications in that section only, unless otherwise stated. FDA = U.S. Food and Drug Administration; GAD = generalized anxiety disorder; SSRI = selective serotonin reuptake inhibitor.

---

tified, for the most part, in individuals with histories of addiction-proneness.

Buspirone, a 5-HT$_{1A}$ agonist nonbenzodiazepine anti-anxiety agent, may have similar efficacy to the benzodiazepines in treating GAD. Its advantages are a different side-effect profile without sedation and the absence of tolerance and withdrawal. Its disadvantage is a slower rate of onset (Rickels et al. 1988), which can lead to early patient noncompliance. Rickels and colleagues compared the efficacy of the benzodiazepine clorazepate to the nonbenzodiazepine buspirone in the acute treatment, maintenance, and discontinuation of patients with GAD (Rickels et al. 1988). The two medications had similar efficacy by the fourth week of treatment, and benefits were maintained during a 6-month period, with an approximately 60% reduction of anxiety scores. There was no evidence of tolerance to either medication during the 6-month period. In the first two weeks of discontinuation of the medications, patients who had been taking clorazepate had a transient increase of anxiety consistent with withdrawal, whereas buspirone patients did not. Treatment with buspirone is usually started at 5 mg tid, and the dose can be increased until a maximum dosage of 60 mg/day is reached. A twice-a-day regimen is probably as efficacious as a three-times-a-day regimen and makes compliance easier. There has been a suggestion in the literature that patients previously treated with benzodiazepines might not respond successfully to buspirone (Schweizer et al. 1986). However, a later controlled double-blind study refuted this suggestion by finding that patients who gradually discontinued the benzodiazepine lorazepam and were then treated with buspirone did not exhibit benzodiazepine withdrawal or rebound anxiety and that they fared as well with buspirone as they had with lorazepam (Delle Chiaie et al. 1995). On the other hand, other researchers (DeMartinis et al. 2000) retrospectively analyzed a large data set with respect to history of benzodiazepine use prior to a controlled clinical trial. They found that clinical response to buspirone was similar to benzodiazepine response in patients who had never used benzodiazepines, but patients who had used benzodiazepines within 1 month of starting the trial had a higher attrition rate and less clinical improvement if by randomization in the study they received buspirone rather than benzodiazepine. There is recent evidence, by way of a controlled trial (Rickels et al. 2000a), that in long-term benzodiazepine users, a successful strategy might be to start buspirone or an antidepressant for 1 month prior to undertaking a gradual 4–6-week taper of the benzodiazepine. Other independent predictors of successful tapering of benzodiazepine were lower initial doses and less severe, less chronic anxiety symptoms.

Antidepressants

Over the past few years, newer antidepressants have become established as first-line treatments for GAD, because there are now controlled trials documenting their efficacy and, in addition, they tend to be well tolerated, require only once-daily dosing, and do not carry a risk of abuse and dependence. Three large, controlled trials have established the efficacy of, and have led to a specific FDA indication for extended-release venlafaxine, an SNRI, in GAD (Davidson et al. 1999; Gelenberg et al. 2000; Rickels et al. 2000b). In two-large placebo-controlled trials, venlafaxine at dosages of 75 mg, 150 mg, and 225 mg/day was found to be effective in treating GAD, in one trial over an 8-week period (Rickels et al. 2000b) and in the other over a 6-month period (Gelenberg et al. 2000). The latter showed an approximately 70% response rate, with benefits appearing as early as the first 2 weeks of treatment. Venlafaxine was generally well tolerated—nausea, somnolence, and dry mouth being the most common side effects. Neither trial showed differences between the doses of venlafaxine, suggesting it can be started at 75mg/day for GAD and subsequently be increased if clinical improvement is not adequate and side effects permit. In another trial comparing venlafaxine 75–150 mg, buspirone 30 mg, and placebo in GAD without depression during an 8-week period, both medications were superior to placebo, and there was weak evidence for possible superiority of venlafaxine over buspirone by some, but not all, measures (Davidson et al. 1999).

In addition to venlafaxine, the SSRI paroxetine has recently been found to be efficacious in treating GAD in a number of controlled studies, findings that have led to a specific FDA indication for this agent in GAD. The first trial (Rocca et al. 1997) found paroxetine 20 mg/day to have similar efficacy to imipramine and benzodiazepine in treating GAD. A large recent trial showed paroxetine at fixed dosages of 20 mg/day or 40 mg/day to be superior to placebo during an 8-week treatment period, with approximately two-thirds of patients considered responders (Bellew et al. 2000). Additionally, a recent, large flexible-dosing trial showed that paroxetine in dosages ranging from 20–50 mg/day was superior to placebo in treating GAD during an 8-week period (Pollack et al. 2001). It also showed that about two-thirds of patients who did not respond to the initial 20-mg dosage responded to higher dosages of 30 mg, 40 mg, or 50 mg/day (McCafferty et al. 2001). Although SSRIs other than paroxetine have not yet been tested in GAD, it is quite possible that they would be efficacious, and trials are under way. Finally, nefazodone was successful in treating GAD in one open trial (Hedges et al. 1996), and mirtazapine in an open trial with comorbid major depression (Goodnick et al. 1999). Some data suggest an early antianxiety response with mirtazapine.

Several older studies have shown TCAs to be effective in treating chronically anxious patients independent of the presence of depressive symptoms, although TCA use has largely fallen out of favor recently in light of the newer antidepressants. In one controlled study comparing imipramine and alprazolam in treating GAD, similar efficacy was found for the two medications, with imipramine acting more on negative affects and cognitions, and alprazolam acting more on somatic symptoms (Hoehn-Saric et al. 1988). In another study, imipramine up to 143 mg/day, trazodone up to 255 mg/day, and diazepam up to 26 mg/day were found comparable after 8 weeks of treatment, with about two-thirds of GAD patients experiencing moderate to marked improvement in anxiety. Not surprisingly, during the first 2 weeks of treatment somatic symptoms responded faster to diazepam (Rickels et al. 1993b).

Other Medications

Beta-adrenergic blocking drugs, such as propranolol, may only be rarely indicated as an adjuvant in patients who experience significant palpitations or tremor. Clonidine, which inhibits locus coeruleus discharge, would seem for theoretical reasons to be a good antianxiety drug. A tendency to lose clinical response, plus a number of bothersome side effects, makes clonidine a poor initial choice for treatment. However, one controlled study found clonidine to be efficacious for both panic disorder and GAD (Hoehn-Saric et al. 1981).

■ SOCIAL PHOBIA

The pharmacological treatment of social phobia is summarized in Table 6–3. A number of medication options can clearly be helpful in social phobia.

Beta-Blockers in Performance Anxiety

In performance-type social phobia, results of several analog studies (i.e., studies using nonclinical samples with performance or social anxiety) have shown beta-blocker efficacy, particularly when these agents are used acutely prior to a performance (Brantigan et al.

TABLE 6–3. **Pharmacological treatment of social phobia**

Selective serotonin reuptake inhibitors

General indications: First-line treatment; shown efficacy; well tolerated; once-daily dosing; effective for comorbid depression, panic, GAD, or OCD

Specific medications

Paroxetine: best-studied in large controlled trials; FDA approved; average dose 40 mg/day

Sertraline: 50–200 mg/day; FDA approved

Citalopram: open trials

Fluoxetine: open trials

Fluvoxamine: smaller controlled trials, average dose 200 mg/day; large, controlled trial with controlled-release formulation

Monoamine oxidase inhibitors

General indications: Demonstrated high effectiveness; may be difficult to tolerate and require dietary restrictions; effective for several comorbid conditions, including atypical depression, social phobia, and panic; well worth trying in patients whose condition is otherwise treatment-refractory

Specific medications

Phenelzine: most studied

Tranylcypromine: also effective

Benzodiazepines

General indications: Clinically widely used and reportedly efficacious in open trials; generally well tolerated; patients need monitoring for dependence and withdrawal symptoms

Specific medications

Clonazepam: long-acting; efficacy demonstrated in controlled trial

Gabapentin

General indications: Found effective in controlled trial, mean dose 2900 mg/day. Consider for augmentation or as second-line treatment if inadequate response to or intolerance for SSRIs

Beta-blockers

General indications: Highly effective for performance anxiety, taken on as-needed basis about 1 hour before event. Usually not helpful in patients with generalized social phobia

TABLE 6–3.   **Pharmacological treatment of social phobia** *(continued)*

Specific medications

    Propranolol

    Atenolol

Other medications

    Buspirone: well tolerated, effective in open trial but not in controlled trial

    Nefazodone: effective in open trial

    Venlafaxine: effective in open trials (use in patients unable to tolerate or unresponsive to SSRIs)

    Bupropion: effective in open trial

    Reversible monoamine oxidase inhibitors: moclobemide: modestly effective to ineffective, not marketed in United States

Note. "FDA approved" refers to approval specifically for use in the disorder named in the table title. Comparisons made in any section on specific medications refer to medications in that section only, unless otherwise stated. FDA = U.S. Food and Drug Administration; GAD = generalized anxiety disorder; OCD = obsessive-compulsive disorder; SSRI = selective serotonin reuptake inhibitor.

1982; Hartley et al. 1983; James et al. 1977; James et al. 1983; Liden and Gottfries 1974; Neftel et al. 1982). Many performing artists or public speakers find that beta-blockers, taken orally a few hours before stage time, reduce palpitations, tremor, and the "butterfly feeling." Although a variety of beta-blockers have been used in studies and are probably efficacious for performance anxiety, the most common ones used are propranolol in doses of approximately 20 mg or atenolol 50 mg, taken about 45 minutes before a performance. It also seems that they are more effective in controlling stage fright, with minimal or no side effects, than are benzodiazepines, which may decrease subjective anxiety, but not optimize performance, and may have an adverse effect on sharpness.

Monoamine Oxidase Inhibitors

Until recently, the MAOIs were the medications most proven effective in treating social phobia. Older studies had shown these drugs to be effective in mixed agoraphobic/social phobic subject samples (Mountjoy et al. 1977; Solyom et al. 1973; Solyom et al. 1981; Tyrer et al. 1973). Liebowitz and colleagues conducted a controlled study (Liebowitz et al. 1992) comparing phenelzine, atenolol, and placebo in the treatment of patients with DSM-III (American Psychiatric Association 1980) social phobia. About two-thirds of patients had a marked response to phenelzine in dosages of 45–90 mg/day, whereas atenolol was not superior to placebo. Tranylcypromine in dosages of 40–60 mg/day was also associated with notable improvement in about 80% of patients with DSM-III social phobia treated openly for 1 year (Versiani et al. 1988). One study (Gelernter et al. 1991) compared cognitive-behavioral group treatment with phenelzine, alprazolam, and placebo. Although all groups improved greatly with treatment, phenelzine tended to be superior in absolute clinical response and decreased impairment. Despite their proven efficacy in social phobia, MAOIs are no longer a first-line treatment, given their dietary and medication restrictions, the potential for hypertensive crises, and their side effects, which are frequently not well tolerated. More recently, there was excitement about the possibility that reversible inhibitors of monoamine oxidase (RIMAs), not yet marketed in the United States, might replace MAOIs in the treatment of social phobia, because they are better tolerated and do not require dietary restrictions. However, findings have been disappointing, and several studies have now shown that one of the RIMAs, moclobemide, is at best very modestly effective, or even ineffective, in social phobia (The International Multicenter Clinical Trial Group on Moclobemide in Social Phobia 1997; Noyes et al. 1997; Schneier et al. 1998).

Benzodiazepines

Traditionally, benzodiazepines have also held promise and have been used in treating generalized social phobia, despite the usual concerns about their use. Several open trials have reported positive results; and in one controlled study, clonazepam at dosages of 0.5–3.0 mg/day (mean dosage 2.4 mg/day) was found to be superior to placebo, with a response rate of 78% and with improvement in social anxiety, avoidance, performance, and negative self-evaluation (Davidson et al. 1993). Alprazolam was also found to be superior to placebo, with comparable results to phenelzine and cognitive-behavioral therapy. However, study participants in the alprazolam group had the highest relapse rate 2 months after treatment discontinuation (Gelernter et al. 1991). Given its longer half-life, clonazepam is a better choice than alprazolam. Both have advantages, such as relatively rapid onset of action and good tolerability. Disadvantages are the potential for abuse, withdrawal, relapse, and lack of efficacy for comorbid depression. The benzodiazepines would not be considered a first-line treatment for social phobia.

Selective Serotonin Reuptake Inhibitors

In the past several years, newer antidepressants have been tested and have shown efficacy in treating social phobia, resulting in the SSRIs becoming the first-line treatment for the disorder. Although investigated to varying degrees, there is no reason to believe that SSRIs differ from each other in their efficacy in social phobia; they are generally well tolerated, are easy to dispense and monitor, and are used in standard doses comparable to those used in depression. Paroxetine is now FDA approved for treating social phobia, with efficacy shown in two controlled trials (Baldwin et al. 1999; Stein et al. 1998) in which about one-half to two-thirds of patients were responders to acute treatment, at average dosages of about 40 mg/day. In one controlled trial, fluvoxamine 150 mg/day for 12 weeks resulted in substantial improvement in 46% of patients compared with 7% improvement in the placebo group (van Vliet et al. 1994); these results were supported in a subsequent larger study with a comparable mean dosage of 200 mg/day and response rate of 43% (Stein et al. 1999). Of 20 patients treated openly with sertraline for at least 8 weeks, 80% showed some improvement of their social phobia (Van Ameringen et al. 1994), and the efficacy of sertraline was duplicated in one placebo-controlled study at dosages of 50–200 mg/day (Katzelnick et al. 1995). A very recent large 20-week trial of sertraline versus placebo confirmed the efficacy of the drug, with flexible dosing up to 200 mg/day and a 53% response rate (Van Ameringen et al. 2001). This finding led to FDA approval of sertraline for social phobia. A similar response rate was found in an open trial of fluoxetine (Van Ameringen et al. 1993) and an open trial of citalopram (Bouwer and Stein 1998).

Other Medications

Additional options seem to hold some promise in treating social phobia. Buspirone, a 5-HT$_{1A}$ agonist, initially appeared promising in an open trial (Schneier et al. 1993), but a subsequent controlled trial did not show efficacy (van Vliet et al. 1997). It is conceivable that dosages higher than the 30 mg/day used in the latter trial might have been more beneficial. An open trial of nefazodone revealed some treatment efficacy (Van Ameringen et al. 1999), and this drug may be a good option for patients who cannot tolerate SSRIs. Similarly, two small open trials of venlafaxine—interestingly, in patients for whom SSRIs had not been effective—reported clinical improvement (Altamura et al. 1999; Kelsey 1995). Bupropion is the least-studied antidepressant, but it may have some efficacy in social phobia (Emmanuel et al. 1991). Finally, the anticonvulsant gabapentin belongs to another class of medication that has been studied in a controlled setting and therefore merits serious consideration as a second-line treatment if SSRIs are ineffective or not tolerated. Although gabapentin has not yet been directly compared with SSRIs, alone or as augmentation, a placebo-controlled trial found gabapentin to be superior to placebo at a mean dosage of about 2900 mg/day, with a response rate approaching 40% of subjects (Pande et al. 1999).

■ SPECIFIC PHOBIA

Medications have not been shown to be effective in treating specific phobia. TCAs, benzodiazepines, and beta-blockers generally do not appear useful for treatment of specific phobia, based on the limited number of studies available. One recent, very small controlled trial—in which 11 patients were randomly assigned to either placebo or paroxetine at dosages up to 20 mg/day for 4 weeks—showed that one out of six patients responded to placebo and three out of five to paroxetine (Benjamin et al. 2000). Further trials of serotonergic agents may be warranted.

■ OBSESSIVE-COMPULSIVE DISORDER

Advances of the past 2 decades in the pharmacotherapy of OCD have been quite dramatic and have generated a great deal of excitement for successful treatment of this disorder. What was previously thought to be a rare, psychodynamically laden, and difficult-to-treat illness now appears to have a strong biological component and to respond well to potent serotonin reuptake inhibitors. The pharmacological treatment approach to OCD is summarized in Table 6–4.

Clomipramine

The first extensively studied medication for the treatment of OCD is clomipramine, a potent serotonin reuptake inhibitor with weak norepinephrine reuptake blockade. A series of well-controlled double-blind studies have undisputedly documented the efficacy of clomipramine in reducing OCD symptoms (Ananth et al. 1981; Flament et al. 1985; Insel et al. 1983; Thorén et al. 1980). The largest of these was a multicenter trial comparing clomipramine with placebo in over 500 patients with OCD, a trial that led to FDA approval for this treatment. On an average dosage of 200–250 mg/day of clomipramine, the average reduction in OCD symptoms was about 40%, and about 60% of all patients were clinically much improved or very much improved (Clomipramine Collaborative Study Group 1991). The very low placebo response rate of 2% documents that OCD is a chronic disorder with infrequent spontaneous remissions. Patients should typically start with 25 mg of clomipramine at bedtime, and the dose is then gradually increased by 25 mg every 4 days, or 50 mg every week, until a maximum dose of 250 mg is

TABLE 6–4.   **Pharmacological treatment of obsessive-compulsive disorder**

Serotonin reuptake inhibitors

General indications: First-line treatments; moderate to high doses

Specific medications

Fluoxetine, fluvoxamine, paroxetine, sertraline: efficacy shown in large controlled trials

Citalopram: less studied, efficacy similar to that of other SSRIs

Clomipramine: efficacy shown in multiple controlled trials; may have slight superiority over SSRIs; typically not used until at least two SSRIs have failed secondary to side-effect profile; can be used in low doses in combination with SSRIs in treatment-refractory OCD. Clomipramine and desmethylclomipramine levels must be closely followed for toxicity

Augmentation

General indications: Partial response to serotonin reuptake inhibitors; presence of other target symptoms

Specific medications

Pimozide: comorbid tic disorders or comorbid schizotypal personality

Haloperidol: comorbid tic disorders or comorbid schizotypal personality

Risperidone: effective augmentation in controlled trial, regardless of tics or schizotypy

Olanzapine: effective in open and controlled trial

Pindolol: effective in controlled trial

Clonazepam: effective in controlled trial for comorbid very high anxiety

Buspirone: one positive trial, three negative

Lithium: ineffective in controlled trial

Trazodone: ineffective in controlled trial

MAOIs: hardly any evidence of antiobsessional efficacy; possibly *phenelzine* for symmetry obsessions

Other medications

Intravenous clomipramine: efficacy in controlled trial for treatment-refractory OCD

Plasma exchange and intravenous immunoglobulin: effective in children with streptococcus-related OCD (PANDAS)

Note.   MAOI = monoamine oxidase inhibitor; OCD = obsessive-compulsive disorder; SSRI = selective serotonin reuptake inhibitor; PANDAS = pediatric autoimmune neuropsychiatric disorder associated with streptococcal infections.

reached. Some patients are unable to tolerate the highest dose and may be stabilized at 150–200 mg. Improvement with clomipramine is relatively slow, with maximal effectiveness occurring after 5–12 weeks of treatment. Some of the more common side effects reported by patients are dry mouth, tremor, sedation, nausea, and ejaculatory failure in men. The seizure risk for dosages up to 250 mg/day is comparable to that of other TCAs and acceptable in the absence of prior neurological history. Clomipramine is equally effective for OCD patients with pure obsessions and those with rituals—in contrast to behavioral treatments, which are less useful for patients with obsessions predominantly. Although one study found a greater effect of clomipramine compared with placebo only in the most depressed subgroup (Marks et al. 1980), the majority of studies have found strong specific antiobsessive effects irrespective of depressive symptoms (Ananth et al. 1981; Clomipramine Collaborative Study Group 1991; Flament et al. 1985; Insel et al. 1983; Thorén et al. 1980). Controlled studies have also demonstrated that clomipramine is effective in treating OCD when other antidepressants, such as amitriptyline, nortriptyline, desipramine, and the MAOI clorgyline, have no therapeutic effect (Ananth et al. 1981; Insel et al. 1983; Leonard et al. 1989; Thorén et al. 1980; Zohar and Insel 1987). This finding strongly suggests that improvement in OCD symptoms is mediated through the blockade of serotonin reuptake.

Selective Serotonin Reuptake Inhibitors

Studies with the more selective serotonin reuptake inhibitors have further supported the hypothesis that improvement in OCD symptoms is mediated through the blockade of serotonin reuptake. SSRIs have turned out to be essentially as efficacious as clomipramine. Four SSRIs (fluoxetine, fluvoxamine, sertraline, and paroxetine) have FDA indications for OCD, and two (fluvoxamine and sertraline) have indication in pediatric OCD. A controlled study comparing clomipramine and fluoxetine in OCD did not find a significant difference in efficacy between the two drugs (Pigott et al. 1990), although the fluoxetine response appeared somewhat less robust than the response with clomipramine. Additionally, fluvoxamine and clomipramine have been found to have similar efficacy in treating OCD (Mundo et al. 2000). Numerous large controlled trials emerged in the 1990s, well documenting the efficacy of all SSRIs for this disorder. Fluoxetine has been shown to be superior to placebo in treating OCD, in dosages of 20–60 mg/day, with greater efficacy at higher dosages (Montgomery et al. 1993; Tollefson et al. 1994). Similarly, fluoxetine has been shown to be safe and efficacious in treating OCD in children (Riddle et al. 1992).

Fluvoxamine has also been found to have a notable antiobsessive effect in several controlled studies (Goodman et al. 1989; 1990b; Jenike et al. 1990a; Perse et al. 1987), with efficacy comparable to clomipramine (Freeman et al. 1994; Koran et al. 1996). Goodman and his group showed that fluvoxamine is superior to desipramine in treating OCD, with 52% of patients demonstrating marked clinical improvement independent of initial depression (Goodman et al. 1990b). The required daily dosage is titrated up to a maximum of 300 mg. The controlled-release formulation of fluvoxamine has also been shown to have documented efficacy in OCD (Hollander et al., in press, a). The efficacy of fluvoxamine for OCD has also been demonstrated for adolescents, in dosages of 100–300 mg/day (Apter et al. 1994). The efficacy of fluvoxamine in treating pediatric OCD, ages 8–17, was further confirmed in a multicenter trial using dosages of 50–200 mg/day. Forty-two percent of the study subjects were responders, defined as having a 25% symptomatic improvement, and the medication was well tolerated in the pediatric group; asthenia and insomnia were the most common side effects (Riddle et al. 2001).

Sertraline is another serotonin reuptake inhibitor whose efficacy for OCD has been established. Although an initial placebo-controlled study revealed no beneficial effect (Jenike et al. 1990b), subsequent studies have shown sertraline to be superior to placebo, at dosages ranging from 50 to 200 mg/day (Chouinard 1992; Greist et al. 1995a; Kronig et al. 1999). Response began to appear as early as the third week of treatment and was firmly apparent by the eighth week (Kronig et al. 1999). Similarly, in a large multicenter trial, sertraline in dosages up to 200 mg/day was found to be effective in treating childhood OCD in persons ages 6–17 years. Again, improvement started to appear about the third week, and 42% of children were significantly improved after 12 weeks. The medication was overall well tolerated, the most common side effects being agitation, insomnia, nausea, and tremor (March et al. 1998).

Paroxetine has been shown, at dosages of 40 mg/day and 60 mg/day, to be superior to placebo in OCD. This improvement continues over an additional 6-month extension, and following double-blind discontinuation, relapse rates are notably lower with paroxetine compared with placebo (Hollander et al., in press, b). Citalopram has not been as extensively studied in the treatment of adult OCD, but it too appears to be efficacious. In pediatric OCD, both paroxetine (Rosenberg et al. 1999) and citalopram (Thomsen 1997) were found to be effective and safe in open trials.

Although clomipramine appears to have an edge in documented efficacy for treating OCD in meta-analytic studies, satisfactory systematic comparisons of the various serotonin reuptake inhibitors, balancing benefits and side effects, have not been conducted. Given the similar efficacy of these five medications for OCD, an extremely large prospective study would have to be undertaken in order to demonstrate small but important differences between the various medications. Three meta-analytic studies have addressed these questions by retrospective analyses of treatment data from past trials, and these have supported a small but important superiority for clomipramine over the SSRIs (Greist et al. 1995b; Piccinelli et al. 1995; Stein et al. 1995). The clinical applicability of this finding may however, in reality, be limited, because in clinical practice, actual or expected tolerability of different medications often takes precedence over small differences in efficacy. The SSRIs are better tolerated than clomipramine by most patients, because of clomipramine's strong anticholinergic side effects, and have therefore become the well-established first line of treatment for OCD. If patients do not have a good response to an adequate trial of at least two SSRIs, augmentation with clomipramine or switching to clomipramine alone should be undertaken; the reverse is also true. The SNRI venlafaxine has also been shown to be effective in small trials of OCD and SSRI-resistant OCD (Ravizza et al. 1995).

Augmentation Strategies

It is important to keep in mind that the medication response in OCD is not as dramatic as in, for example, major depression; a considerable number of patients show a negligible or a partial response to the first-line medications. As a helpful rule of thumb, it is useful to remember that approximately 40%–60% of OCD patients improve by about 30%–60% with a first-line drug. Thus, various combination and augmentation strategies are often needed to attain a satisfactory response. The most commonly used augmenting agents—unfortunately, often without strong scientific findings supporting their effectiveness—are buspirone, lithium, tryptophan, trazodone, clonazepam, risperidone, olanzapine, pindolol, desipramine, and inositol. As these augmentation strategies have come to be more rigorously tested in recent years, many of them, with the exception of the atypical risperidone or olanzapine, do not look as promising as was initially thought. Still, given the relatively limited treatment options, these strategies are well worth undertaking sequentially, beginning with the most compelling ones. The findings in favor or against the various augmenting agents for OCD are summarized below.

Although an initial small study reported similar efficacy for clomipramine alone versus buspirone alone in treating OCD (Pato et al. 1991), three other studies failed to show a significant benefit to buspirone augmentation in patients treated with clomipramine (Pigott et al. 1992a), fluoxetine (Grady et al. 1993), or fluvoxamine (McDougle et al. 1993b). If tried, higher dosages of 30–60 mg/day should be the goal. Controlled study of lithium augmentation of SSRIs did not detect any benefit (McDougle et al. 1991a; Pigott et al. 1991). A controlled study of trazodone alone in OCD again showed no benefit compared with placebo (Pigott et al. 1992b). A controlled crossover study showed clonazepam to be effective in 40% of OCD clomipramine-study subjects not helped by clomipramine (Hewlett et al. 1992); clonazepam may also be helpful with the very high anxiety levels frequently associated with OCD. Evidence in support of MAOI therapy is very weak despite a positive report (Vallejo et al. 1992), possibly with the exception of some benefit from phenelzine for symmetry obsessions (Jenike et al. 1997). A trazodone controlled trial (Pigott et al. 1992b), and a desipramine controlled augmentation trial (Barr et al. 1997) were negative. In a small open trial, 10 OCD patients in serotonin reuptake inhibitor trials who had not been helped by these drugs were treated with inositol augmentation, at 18 mg/day for 6 weeks; only three patients reported clinically significant improvement, leaving inositol an option of unclear efficacy (Seedat and Stein 1999).

Antipsychotics make up a major medication class that can be successfully used to augment partial response to serotonin reuptake inhibitors in OCD. McDougle and colleagues first reported that about 50% of OCD patients improved noticeably when pimozide was added to fluvoxamine (McDougle et al. 1990); comorbid tic disorders or schizotypal personality predicted a good response, supporting the hypothesis that the dopaminergic system may be dysregulated in at least a subgroup of patients with OCD (Goodman et al. 1990a). OCD patients with comorbid tic disorders may actually be less responsive to SSRI monotherapy (McDougle et al. 1993a) and appear to respond well to haloperidol augmentation (McDougle et al. 1994). In more recent years, atypical antipsychotics have received increasing attention as a major augmentation strategy for OCD, regardless of comorbid tics or schizotypy, and this strategy is now supported by controlled trials. Risperidone has been successfully used for augmentation in open trials, with good results for horrific mental imagery rather than comorbid tic disorders (Saxena et al. 1996). In an open 8-week trial, in which risperidone 3 mg/day was added to an SSRI in 20 patients with refractory OCD, all patients were described as showing some improvement (Pfanner et al. 2000). More compelling, a controlled trial of 6-week risperidone in patients refractory to a serotonin reuptake inhibitor found significant improvement in one-half of the patients (McDougle et al. 2000); this response was not associated with whether or not tics or schizotypy were present. Four pediatric patients with refractory OCD have also been described as responsive to risperidone augmentation (Fitzgerald et al. 1999). Olanzapine appears as promising as does risperidone. In a 3-month open augmentation trial with olanzapine in OCD patients who had not responded to fluvoxamine, almost one-half showed notable improvement (Bogetto et al. 2000). Similarly, benefits were noted in the majority of subjects with partial response to an SSRI augmented openly with olanzapine for 8 weeks (Weiss et al. 1999). In a sample of nine OCD patients whose condition was refractory to treatment and for whom three trials using serotonin-reuptake inhibitors had shown no improvement, three showed at least a 30% improvement with 8-week open olanzapine augmentation at dosages of 2.5–10.0 mg/day (Koran et al. 2000). In considering antipsychotics, one should note that the atypical antipsychotic clozapine has been reported to worsen OCD when used as monotherapy (Baker et al. 1992; Ghaemi et al. 1995).

Other than antipsychotics, pindolol is the only additional medication that has proven a useful augmentation agent in a controlled study (Dannon et al. 2000). Fourteen patients with treatment-refractory OCD whose condition had not improved in three SSRI trials received paroxetine augmentation with pindolol or placebo for 6 weeks. Compared with placebo, pindolol at 2.5 mg tid was notably superior in reducing OCD symptoms.

The combination of clomipramine with an SSRI is also a commonly used strategy for treating patients whose OCD is refractory to treatment, and the combination is generally well tolerated. However, lower doses of clomipramine than would be prescribed if taken independently should be used—and blood levels should be monitored—to avoid toxicity, because clomipramine levels can become markedly elevated (Szegedi et al. 1996). In one small, randomized trial in patients with treatment-refractory OCD, citalopram combined with clomipramine led to much greater improvement than citalopram alone (Pallanti et al. 1999).

Treatment of Refractory Obsessive-Compulsive Disorder

When oral medications fail to be successful enough in patients with highly refractory OCD, other options can be considered—including, of course, cognitive-behavioral techniques, described in Chapter 7 (if these have not already been instituted), as well as a number of other biological interventions. Electroconvulsive therapy may also be considered in highly refractory conditions, although its efficacy is debatable (Maletzky et al. 1994). Intravenous clomipramine has met with success in some patients whose OCD is treatment-refractory to oral clomipramine (Fallon et al. 1992; Warneke 1985). In a more recent controlled study, intravenous clomipramine proved more effective than intravenous placebo in a trial of 54 OCD patients whose condition was refractory to oral clomipramine; 58% of the 54 study participants experienced fewer and less intense refractory symptoms, and the treatment was safely tolerated (Fallon et al. 1998). Plasma exchange and intravenous immunoglobulin have been found to be effective in lessening the severity of symptoms in children with streptococcal-infection–triggered OCD (Perlmutter et al. 1999), but plasma exchange treatment was found not to help children whose OCD did not have streptococcus-related exacerbations (Nicolson et al. 2000).

In extreme cases of treatment-refractory OCD in severely impaired patients, neurosurgery can be considered. In a thorough retrospective analysis, Jenike and his group (Jenike et al.1991) estimated that in at least 25%–30% of patients, cingulotomy resulted in notable improvement. This response rate was confirmed in a 2-year prospective cingulotomy study (Baer et al. 1995). A comparable response rate of 38% was reported in another study at 10 years of follow-up after the stereotactic surgery (Hay et al. 1993). Guidelines for the use of neurosurgical techniques in the treatment of severe, refractory OCD, including selection, documented failed treatments, indications, contraindications, benefits and risks, and workup have been thoroughly reviewed elsewhere (Mindus and Jenike 1992). A recent review of 29 patients who underwent capsulotomy between 1976 and 1989 at the Karolinska Hospital (Stockholm, Sweden) found that successful lesioning localized to the middle of the anterior limb of the internal capsule (Lippitz et al. 1999). Gamma knife surgery and deep brain stimulation are currently under study in OCD. Most recently, transcranial magnetic stimulation has been tried in OCD and appears to have some promise, but the topic requires much further study (Greenberg et al. 1997).

Predictors and Course of Treatment

Although there are no definitive predictors of response to medication treatment, several factors appear to be predictive of a poorer prognosis: earlier age at onset, longer duration of illness, greater frequency of compulsions, washing rituals, a chronic course, prior hospitalizations, and the presence of avoidant, borderline, or schizotypal personality disorder, as well as of more than one personality disorder (Ackerman et al. 1994; Baer and Jenike 1992; Baer et al. 1992; Ravizza et al. 1995). A review of 274 patients with OCD has recently found no differences between responsive and non-responsive study subjects in age, gender, age at onset, duration of illness, or symptom subtypes. Responsive patients had a higher incidence of family history of tics, sudden onset of OCD, and an episodic course of illness. Nonresponsive patients had more severe symptomatology, poorer insight into their OCD, and comorbid eating disorder (Hollander et al. 2001).

OCD tends to be a chronic illness, and many patients require long-term medication to stay well. Generally, long-term continuation of medication treatment maintains a good response to treatment; this premise is widely supported in clinical treatment and has been validated by a 1-year double-blind sertraline maintenance study with maintenance dosages of 50–200 mg/day (Greist et al. 1995c). In a subsequent study, patients who maintained their response in the Greist study were given a second year of open maintenance treatment with sertraline at the same dosages, during which they maintained or even slightly improved their gains (Rasmussen et al. 1997). Conversely, in a double-blind discontinuation study of

OCD patients who had done well taking clomipramine for about 1 year, 90% worsened substantially within 7 weeks when the medication was discontinued (Pato et al. 1988). The same relapse rate of 90% was found in an adolescent OCD group when chronic clomipramine was blindly substituted with 8 weeks of desipramine (Leonard et al. 1991). Again at 1-year follow-up, patients who were randomly assigned to continue fluoxetine rather than be switched to placebo had much lower rates of relapse (Romano et al. 2001). At follow-up after several years, most patients remain symptomatic and require continued pharmacotherapy; in a substantial minority (20%) the condition remains refractory to multiple treatment regimens (Leonard et al. 1993).

■ POSTTRAUMATIC STRESS DISORDER

A variety of different psychopharmacological agents have been used in the treatment of posttraumatic stress disorder (PTSD) by clinicians and have been reported in the literature as case reports, open clinic trials, and controlled studies. These agents are presented below and summarized in Table 6–5. In the past several years, SSRIs and other serotonergic agents have emerged as the first-line pharmacological treatment of PTSD.

Adrenergic Blockers

Kolb and colleagues treated 12 Vietnam War veterans with PTSD in an open trial of the beta-blocker propranolol during a 6-month period (Kolb et al. 1984). Dosage ranged from 120 mg/day to 160 mg/day. Eleven of the study participants reported positive changes on self-assessment at the end of the 6-month period, including less explosiveness; fewer nightmares; improved sleep; and a decrease in intrusive thoughts, hyperalertness, and startle reactions. Another open pilot study by this group (Kolb et al. 1984), using clonidine, a noradrenergic alpha-agonist, was conducted with 9 Vietnam War veterans with PTSD. Clonidine dosages of 0.2–0.4 mg/day was administered during a 6-month period. Eight patients reported

TABLE 6–5. **Pharmacological treatment of posttraumatic stress disorder**

Selective serotonin reuptake inhibitors

General indications: First-line treatment; well tolerated; once/day dosing; documented efficacy

Specific medications

    Sertraline: FDA approved, large controlled trials

    Paroxetine: FDA approved

    Fluoxetine: large controlled trials

    Fluvoxamine: open trials, similar efficacy

    Citalopram: open trials, similar efficacy

Nefazodone

General indications: Next first-line option if poor response to or intolerance of SSRIs; several open trials, one in patients with treatment-refractory disorder; no controlled trials

Other antidepressants

    Tricyclic antidepressants: overall modest results when tested in double-blind study design

    MAOIs: may be superior to tricyclic antidepressants, especially for intrusive symptoms

Augmentation

General indications: When response to first-line options not adequate and as additional treatment of specific PTSD symptoms or comorbid disorders

    Clonidine: some efficacy shown in open treatment; used for nightmares and flashbacks

    Lithium: improvement in intrusive symptoms and irritability shown in open trial

    Carbamazepine: decrease intrusive symptoms, anger, impulsivity in open treatment

    Valproic acid: decreased hyperarousal and intrusion, not numbing, shown in open treatment

    Lamotrigine: very small controlled trial, some efficacy

    Buspirone: efficacy in an open trial

    Triiodothyronine: improvement in small open trial, possibly via an antidepressant response

    Cyproheptadine: case reports of decreased nightmares

TABLE 6–5.	**Pharmacological treatment of posttraumatic stress disorder** *(continued)*

Bupropion: no change in PTSD but improvement in depression shown in open treatment

Trazodone: used for sleep disturbance

Prazosin: shown more effective than placebo for PTSD symptoms, especially for nightmares and sleep disturbance

Benzodiazepines: sleep disturbance

Diphenhydramine: sleep disturbance

Note. Comparisons made in any section on specific medications refer to medications in that section only, unless otherwise stated. FDA = U.S. Food and Drug Administration; MAOI = monoamine oxidase inhibitor; PTSD = posttraumatic stress disorder; SSRI = selective serotonin reuptake inhibitor.

improvements in their capacity to control their emotions and in lessened explosiveness. A majority reported improvements in sleep and nightmares; lowered startle, hyperalertness, and intrusive thinking; and psychosocial improvement. These findings support the role of noradrenergic hyperactivity in the maintenance of autonomic arousal symptoms in PTSD. In a retrospective treatment review of Cambodian patients with PTSD, Kinzie and Leung (1989) found that the majority of patients benefited from the combination of clonidine and a TCA, as opposed to either medication taken alone. Controlled studies of adrenergic blockers in PTSD are needed.

Tricyclic Antidepressants

Until about a decade ago, most reports on the pharmacotherapy of PTSD involved the use of TCAs. A retrospective study by Bleich and colleagues of 25 PTSD patients treated with a variety of different antidepressants, including TCAs and MAOIs, reported good or moderate results in 67% of cases treated (Bleich et al. 1986). Response was not clearly related to the presence of somatization symptoms, depression, or panic attacks. Antidepressants appeared to be more useful than major tranquilizers. Antidepressants improved intrusion symptoms, but the most prominent general effects were alleviation of insomnia and overall sedation. Antidepressants were also found to have a positive effect on psychotherapy in 70% of cases.

Burstein (1984), in administering imipramine in dosages of 50–350 mg/day to 10 patients with PTSD of recent onset, observed significant improvement in intrusive recollections, sleep and dream disturbance, and flashbacks. Similar improvement in intrusive symptoms was reported with an open trial of desipramine (Kauffman et al. 1987). A positive effect of imipramine on posttraumatic night terrors was reported by Marshall (1975).

Later, controlled studies of TCAs in PTSD were conducted but, overall, did not replicate the success in decreasing posttraumatic symptoms reported in earlier trials. In a 4-week, double-blind crossover study of desipramine and placebo in 18 veterans with PTSD, only depressive symptoms improved; anxiety, intrusive symptoms, and avoidance did not change with desipramine therapy (Reist et al. 1989). Davidson and colleagues conducted a 4–8 week double-blind comparison (Davidson et al. 1990) of amitriptyline and placebo in 46 veterans with PTSD. Although depression and anxiety decreased, decrease in intrusive and avoidant symptoms was apparent only in a subgroup of patients who completed 8 weeks of amitriptyline, and that decrease was minimal. At the end of the study, roughly two-thirds of patients in both treatment groups still met criteria for PTSD.

Monoamine Oxidase Inhibitors

An early study of MAOIs described five patients with "traumatic war neurosis" in whom phenelzine, in dosages of 45–75 mg/day, improved symptoms including traumatic dreams, flashbacks, startle reactions, and violent outbursts (Hogben and Cornfield 1981). Panic attacks were also described in all of the patients in this study. Positive effects of phenelzine on intrusive posttraumatic symptoms have been reported in subsequent small open trials (Davidson et al. 1987; van der Kolk 1983).

Subsequently, an 8-week randomized double-blind trial compared phenelzine (71 mg), imipramine (240 mg), and placebo in 34 veterans with PTSD (Frank et al. 1988). Both antidepressants resulted in some overall improvement in patients' posttraumatic symptoms, and phenelzine tended to be superior to imipramine. The most marked improvement was the decrease in intrusive symptoms in patients taking phenelzine, with 60% average reduction on the intrusion scale measure.

Selective Serotonin Reuptake Inhibitors

Earlier, multiple open trials with SSRIs suggested that these medications had at least modest efficacy for the treatment of PTSD, and in the past few years SSRIs have become the medications of choice for this disorder. Several initial open trials of fluoxetine had reported marked improvement in PTSD symptoms at a wide range of doses (Davidson et al. 1991; McDougle et al. 1991b; Shay 1992). Subsequently, in a double-blind trial comparing fluoxetine and placebo, fluoxetine led to a significant reduction of PTSD symptomatology, especially for arousal and numbing symptoms (van der Kolk et al. 1994). An initial open trial of sertraline (Brady et al. 1995) had also claimed benefit for PTSD. Sertraline is now FDA approved for the treatment of PTSD, after two large controlled trials recently documented its efficacy. In a 12-week multicenter placebo-controlled trial, sertraline at dosages of 50–200 mg/day resulted in notable benefits, which began to appear by week 2. The response rate among study participants was greater than 50%, and improvement in both numbing and arousal symptoms (but not reexperiencing) was much greater than with placebo (Brady et al. 2000). Very similar results were reported in another large sertraline study with very similar design (Davidson et al. 2001), with a 60% responder rate based on conservative intent-to-treat analysis. Open trials of other SSRIs, such as fluvoxamine (De Boer et al. 1992), paroxetine (Marshall et al. 1998), and citalopram (Seedat et al. 2000, 2001) suggest similar efficacy in PTSD. Paroxetine has received an FDA approval for use in PTSD.

Mood Stabilizers and Anticonvulsants

In a small open trial of lithium in treating PTSD, van der Kolk (1983) reported improvement in intrusive recollections and irritability in over half of the patients treated. However, there have been no controlled trials. In an open trial of carbamazepine in 10 patients with PTSD, Lipper and his group (Lipper et al. 1986) reported moderate to great improvement in intrusive symptoms in 7 patients. Wolf and associates reported decreased impulsivity and angry outbursts in 10 veterans who were also treated with carbamazepine (Wolf et al. 1988); all patients had normal results on electroencephalograms (EEGs). Valproic acid was initially reported to decrease irritability and angry outbursts in 2 veterans with PTSD (Szymanski and Olympia 1991). More recently, in an open trial of 16 patients treated with divalproex sodium for 8 weeks, a notable decrease in hyperarousal and intrusion symptoms, but not numbing, was reported (Clark et al. 1999a). In a very small, placebo-controlled trial of lamotrigine at dosages up to 500 mg/day, more patients appeared to respond to lamotrigine (Hertzberg et al. 1999), warranting larger studies.

Other Medications

Several open trials have described benefits with nefazodone treatment. A 12-week study using a mean dosage of 430 mg/day showed improvement in all three symptom clusters in patients with previously treatment-refractory PTSD (Zisook et al. 2000). An 8-week open trial reported similar improvements in chronic PTSD patients (Davis et al. 2000), and another report found a 60% response rate in study participants who completed treatment (Davidson et al. 1998); yet another report described improvement in all of 10 patients treated (Hertzberg et al. 1998). Thus, nefazodone appears very promising in treating PTSD, and a controlled trial is warranted.

A small open trial of buspirone reported that 7 of 8 patients experienced a significant reduction in PTSD symptoms; there are no controlled studies (Duffy and Malloy 1994). In a small open trial, triiodothyronine was reported to result in significant clinical improvement in 4 of 5 PTSD patients who had only partial responses to SSRIs; however, it remains unclear whether or not this was primarily an antidepressant response (Agid et al. 2001). Cyproheptadine has been reported to much decrease the nightmares characteristic of PTSD (Clark et al. 1999b; Gupta et al. 1998). An open trial of bupropion in PTSD reported comprehensive improvement secondary to decreased depression, but PTSD symptoms remained mostly unchanged (Canive et al. 1998).

An interesting recent trial has reported efficacy for prazosin, a centrally active alpha$_1$ adrenergic antagonist, compared to placebo, in reducing PTSD symptoms (Raskind et al. 2002). Specifically, eight Vietnam combat veterans with PTSD were treated with prazosin in a double-blind, placebo-controlled crossover study at a mean dosage of 10 mg/day. All eight subjects showed overall moderate to marked improvement in PTSD while taking the prazosin, with most pronounced effectiveness for nightmares and sleep disturbance.

Other Somatic Treatments

Transcranial magnetic stimulation was found to have some transient efficacy in decreasing core PTSD symptoms in 10 patients treated openly; this technique in PTSD may warrant more investigation (Grisaru et al. 1998).

■ REFERENCES

Ackerman DL, Greenland S, Bystritsky A, et al: Predictors of treatment response in obsessive-compulsive disorder: multivariate analyses from a multicenter trial of clomipramine. J Clin Psychopharmacol 14:247–254, 1994

Agid O, Shalev AY, Lerer B: Triiodothyronine augmentation of selective serotonin reuptake inhibitors in posttraumatic stress disorder. J Clin Psychiatry 62:169–173, 2001

Altamura AC, Pioli R, Vitto M, et al: Venlafaxine in social phobia: a study in selective serotonin reuptake inhibitor non-responders. Int Clin Psychopharmacol 14:239–245, 1999

American Psychiatric Association: Diagnostic and Statistical Manual of Mental Disorders, 3rd Edition. Washington, DC, American Psychiatric Association, 1980

Ananth J, Pecknold JC, Van Den Steen N, et al: Double-blind comparative study of clomipramine and amitriptyline in obsessive neurosis. Prog Neuropsychopharmacol Biol Psychiatry 5:257–262, 1981

Apter A, Ratzoni G, King RA, et al: Fluvoxamine open-label treatment of adolescent inpatients with obsessive-compulsive disorder or depression. J Am Acad Child Adolesc Psychiatry 33:342–348, 1994

Baer L, Jenike MA. Personality disorders in obsessive-compulsive disorder. Psychiatr Clin North Am 15:803–812, 1992

Baer L, Jenike MA, Black DW, et al: Effect of axis II diagnoses on treatment outcome with clomipramine in 55 patients with obsessive-compulsive disorder. Arch Gen Psychiatry 49:862–866, 1992

Baer L, Rauch SL, Ballantine HT, et al: Cingulotomy for intractable obsessive-compulsive disorder. Prospective long-term follow-up of 18 patients. Arch Gen Psychiatry 52:384–392, 1995

Baker RW, Chengappa KN, Baird JW, et al: Emergence of obsessive compulsive symptoms during treatment with clozapine. J Clin Psychiatry 53:439–442, 1992

Baldwin D, Bobes J, Stein DJ, et al: Paroxetine in social phobia/social anxiety disorder: a randomized, double-blind, placebo-controlled study. Br J Psychiatry 175:120–126, 1999

Ballenger JC, Wheadon DE, Steiner M, et al: Double-blind, fixed-dose, placebo-controlled study of paroxetine in the treatment of panic disorder. Am J Psychiatry 155:36–42, 2000

Barr LC, Goodman WK, Anand A, et al: Addition of desipramine to serotonin reuptake inhibitors in treatment-resistant obsessive-compulsive disorder. Am J Psychiatry 154:1293–1295, 1997

Bellew KM, McCafferty JP, Iyengar M, et al: Paroxetine treatment of GAD: a double-blind, placebo-controlled trial. Paper presented at the annual meeting of the American Psychiatric Association, Chicago, IL, May 2000

Benjamin J, Levine J, Fux M, et al: Double-blind, placebo-controlled, crossover trial of inositol treatment for panic disorder. Am J Psychiatry 152:1084–1086, 1995

Benjamin J, Ben-Zion IZ, Karbofsky E, et al: Double-blind, placebo-controlled study of paroxetine for specific phobia. Psychopharmacology (Berl) 149:194–196, 2000

Bleich A, Siegel B, Garb R, et al: Post-traumatic stress disorder following combat exposure: clinical features and psychopharmacological treatment. Br J Psychiatry 149:365–369, 1986

Bogetto F, Bellino S, Vaschetto P, et al: Olanzapine augmentation of fluvoxamine-refractory obsessive-compulsive disorder (OCD): a 12-week open trial. Psychiatry Res 96:91–98, 2000

Bouwer C, Stein DJ: Use of the selective serotonin reuptake inhibitor citalopram in the treatment of generalized social phobia. J Affect Disord 49:79–82, 1998

Boyer W: Serotonin uptake inhibitors are superior to imipramine and alprazolam in alleviating panic attacks: a meta-analysis. Int Clin Psychopharmacol 10:45–49, 1995

Brady KT, Sonne SC, Roberts JM: Sertraline treatment of comorbid post-traumatic stress disorder and alcohol dependence. J Clin Psychiatry 56:502–505, 1995

Brady K, Pearlstein T, Asnis GM, et al: Efficacy and safety of sertraline treatment of posttraumatic stress disorder: a randomized controlled trial. JAMA 283:1837–1844, 2000

Brantigan CO, Brantigan TA, Joseph N: Effect of beta blockade and beta stimulation on stage fright. Am J Med 72:88–94, 1982

Burstein A: Treatment of post-traumatic stress disorder with imipramine. Psychosomatics 25:681–687, 1984

Caillard V, Rouillon F, Viel JF, et al: Comparative effects of low and high doses of clomipramine and placebo in panic disorder: a double-blind, controlled study. French University Antidepressant Group. Acta Psychiatr Scand 99:51–58, 1999

Canive JM, Clark RD, Calais LA, et al: Bupropion treatment in veterans with posttraumatic stress disorder: an open study. J Clin Psychopharmacol 18:379–383, 1998

Chouinard G: Sertraline in the treatment of obsessive compulsive disorder: two double-blind, placebo-controlled studies. Int Clin Psychopharmacol 7[suppl 2]:37–41, 1992

Clark RD, Canive JM, Calais LA, et al: Divalproex in posttraumatic stress disorder: an open-label clinical trial. J Trauma Stress 12:395–401, 1999a

Clark RD, Canive JM, Calais LA, et al: Cyproheptadine treatment of nightmares associated with posttraumatic stress disorder. J Clin Psychopharmacol 19:486–487, 1999b

Clomipramine Collaborative Study Group: Clomipramine in the treatment of patients with obsessive-compulsive disorder. Arch Gen Psychiatry 48:730–738, 1991

Dannon PN, Sasson Y, Hirschmann S, et al: Pindolol augmentation in treatment-resistant obsessive compulsive disorder: a double-blind placebo controlled trial. Eur Neuropsychopharmacol 10:165–169, 2000

Davidson J, Walker JI, Kilts C: A pilot study of phenelzine in the treatment of post-traumatic stress disorder. Br J Psychiatry 150:252–255, 1987

Davidson J, Kudler H, Smith R, et al: Treatment of posttraumatic stress disorder with amitriptyline and placebo. Arch Gen Psychiatry 47:259–266, 1990

Davidson J, Roth S, Newman E: Fluoxetine in post-traumatic stress disorder. J Trauma Stress 4:419–423, 1991

Davidson J, Potts N, Richichi E, et al: Treatment of social phobia with clonazepam and placebo. J Clin Psychopharmacol 13:423–428, 1993

Davidson JR, Weisler RH, Malik ML, et al: Treatment of posttraumatic stress disorder with nefazodone. Int Clin Psychopharmacol 13:111–113, 1998

Davidson JR, DuPont RL, Hedges D, et al: Efficacy, safety, and tolerability of venlafaxine extended release and buspirone in outpatients with generalized anxiety disorder. J Clin Psychiatry 60:528–535, 1999

Davidson DR, Rothbaum BO, van der Kolk BA, et al: Multicenter, double-blind comparison of sertraline and placebo in the treatment of posttraumatic stress disorder. Arch Gen Psychiatry 58:485–492, 2001

Davis LL, Nugent AL, Murray J, et al: Nefazodone treatment for chronic posttraumatic stress disorder: an open trial. J Clin Psychopharmacol 20:159–164, 2000

De Boer M, Op den Velde W, Falger PJ, et al: Fluvoxamine treatment for chronic PTSD: a pilot study. Psychother Psychosom 57:158–163, 1992

Delle Chiaie R, Pancheri P, Casacchia M, et al: Assessment of the efficacy of buspirone in patients affected by generalized anxiety disorder, shifting to buspirone from prior treatment with lorazepam: a placebo-controlled, double-blind study. J Clin Psychopharmacol 15:12–19, 1995

DeMartinis N, Schweizer E, Rickels K: An open-label trial of nefazodone in high comorbidity panic disorder. J Clin Psychiatry 57:245–248, 1996

DeMartinis N, Rynn M, Rickels K, et al: Prior benzodiazepine use and buspirone response in the treatment of generalized anxiety disorder. J Clin Psychiatry 61:91–94, 2000

Den Boer JA: Serotonergic Mechanisms in Anxiety Disorders: An Inquiry into Serotonin Function in Panic Disorder. The Hague, Netherlands, Cip-Gegevens Koninklijke Bibliotheek, 1988

Duffy JD, Malloy PF: Efficacy of buspirone in the treatment of posttraumatic stress disorder: an open trial. Ann Clin Psychiatry 6:33–37, 1994

Emmanuel NP, Lydiard BR, Ballenger JC: Treatment of social phobia with bupropion. J Clin Psychopharmacol 1:276–277, 1991

Fallon BA, Campeas R, Schneier FR, et al: Open trial of intravenous clomipramine in five treatment-refractory patients with obsessive-compulsive disorder. J Neuropsychiatry Clin Neurosci 4:70–75, 1992

Fallon BA, Liebowitz MR, Campeas R, et al: Intravenous clomipramine for obsessive-compulsive disorder refractory to oral clomipramine: a placebo-controlled study. Arch Gen Psychiatry 55:918–924, 1998

Fitzgerald KD, Stewart CM, Tawile V, et al: Risperidone augmentation of serotonin reuptake inhibitor treatment of pediatric obsessive compulsive disorder. J Child Adolesc Psychopharmacol 9:115–123, 1999

Flament MF, Rapoport JL, Berg CJ, et al: Clomipramine treatment of childhood obsessive-compulsive disorder: a double-blind controlled study. Arch Gen Psychiatry 42:977–983, 1985

Frank JB, Kosten TR, Giller EL Jr, et al: A randomized clinical trial of phenelzine and imipramine for posttraumatic stress disorder. Am J Psychiatry 145:1289–1291, 1988

Freeman CP, Trimble MR, Deakin JF, et al: Fluvoxamine versus clomipramine in the treatment of obsessive compulsive disorder: a multicenter, randomized, double-blinded, parallel group comparison. J Clin Psychiatry 55:301–305, 1994

Gelenberg AJ, Lydiard RB, Rudolph RL, et al: Efficacy of venlafaxine extended-release capsules in nondepressed outpatients with generalized anxiety disorder: a 6-month randomized controlled trial. JAMA 283:3082–3088, 2000

Gelernter CS, Uhde TW, Cimbolic P, et al: Cognitive-behavioral and pharmacological treatments of social phobia: a controlled study. Arch Gen Psychiatry 48:938–945, 1991

Geracioti TD: Venlafaxine treatment of panic disorder: a case series. J Clin Psychiatry 56:408–410, 1995

Ghaemi SN, Zarate CA, Popli AP, et al: Is there a relationship between clozapine and obsessive-compulsive disorder? A retrospective chart review. Compr Psychiatry 36:267–270, 1995

Goddard AW, Brouette T, Almai A, et al: Early coadministration of clonazepam with sertraline for panic disorder. Arch Gen Psychiatry 58:681–686, 2001

Goodman WK, Price LH, Rasmussen SA, et al: Efficacy of fluvoxamine in obsessive-compulsive disorder: a double-blind comparison with placebo. Arch Gen Psychiatry 46:36–44, 1989

Goodman WK, McDougle CJ, Price LH, et al: Beyond the serotonin hypothesis: a role for dopamine in some forms of obsessive compulsive disorder? J Clin Psychiatry 51 (suppl 8):36–43, 1990a

Goodman WK, Price LH, Delgado PL, et al: Specificity of serotonin reuptake inhibitors in the treatment of obsessive-compulsive disorder: comparison of fluoxetine and desipramine. Arch Gen Psychiatry 47:577–585, 1990b

Goodnick PJ, Puig A, DeVane CL, et al: Mirtazapine in major depression with comorbid generalized anxiety disorder. J Clin Psychiatry 60:446–448, 1999

Grady TA, Pigott TA, L'Heureux F, et al: Double-blind study of adjuvant buspirone for fluoxetine-treated patients with obsessive-compulsive disorder. Am J Psychiatry 150:819–821, 1993

Greenberg BD, George MS, Martin JD, et al: Effect of prefrontal repetitive transcranial magnetic stimulation in obsessive-compulsive disorder: a preliminary study. Am J Psychiatry 154:867–869, 1997

Greist J, Chouinard G, DuBoff E, et al: Double-blind parallel comparison of three dosages of sertraline and placebo in outpatients with obsessive-compulsive disorder. Arch Gen Psychiatry 52:289–295, 1995a

Greist JH, Jefferson JW, Kobak KA, et al: Efficacy and tolerability of serotonin transport inhibitors in obsessive-compulsive disorder. A meta-analysis. Arch Gen Psychiatry 52:53–60, 1995b

Greist JH, Jefferson JW, Kobak KA, et al: A 1 year double-blind placebo-controlled fixed dose study of sertraline in the treatment of obsessive-compulsive disorder. Int Clin Psychopharmacol 10:57–65, 1995c

Grisaru N, Amir M, Cohen H, et al: Effect of transcranial magnetic stimulation in posttraumatic stress disorder: a preliminary study. Biol Psychiatry 44:52–55, 1998

Gupta S, Popli A, Bathurst E, et al: Efficacy of cyproheptadine for nightmares associated with posttraumatic stress disorder. Compr Psychiatry 39:160–164, 1998

Hartley LR, Ungapen S, Davie I, et al: The effect of beta adrenergic blocking drugs on speakers' performance and memory. Br J Psychiatry 142:512–517, 1983

Hay P, Sachdev P, Cumming S, et al: Treatment of obsessive-compulsive disorder by psychosurgery. Acta Psychiatr Scand 87:197–207, 1993

Hedges DW, Reimherr FW, Strong RE, et al: An open trial of nefazodone in adult patients with generalized anxiety disorder. Psychopharmacol Bull 32:671–676, 1996

Hertzberg MA, Feldman ME, Beckham JC, et al: Open trial of nefazodone for combat-related posttraumatic stress disorder. J Clin Psychiatry 59:460–464, 1998

Hertzberg MA, Butterfield MI, Feldman ME, et al: A preliminary study of lamotrigine for the treatment of posttraumatic stress disorder. Biol Psychiatry 45:1226–1229, 1999

Hewlett WA, Vinogradov S, Agras WS: Clomipramine, clonazepam, and clonidine treatment of obsessive-compulsive disorder. J Clin Psychopharmacol 12:420–430, 1992

Hirschmann S, Dannon PN, Iancu I, et al: Pindolol augmentation in patients with treatment-resistant panic disorder: a double-blind, placebo-controlled trial. J Clin Psychopharmacol 20:556–559, 2000

Hoehn-Saric R, Merchant AF, Keyser ML, et al: Effects of clonidine on anxiety disorders. Arch Gen Psychiatry 38:1278–1282, 1981

Hoehn-Saric R, McLeod DR, Zimmerli WD: Differential effects of alprazolam and imipramine in generalized anxiety disorder: somatic versus psychic symptoms. J Clin Psychiatry 49:293–301, 1988

Hoehn-Saric R, McLeod DR, Hipsley PA: Effect of fluvoxamine on panic disorder. J Clin Psychopharmacol 13:321–326, 1993

Hogben GL, Cornfield RB: Treatment of traumatic war neurosis with phenelzine. Arch Gen Psychiatry 38:440–445, 1981

Hollander E, Bienstock C, Pallanti S, et al: The International Treatment Refractory OCD Consortium: preliminary findings. Paper presented at the Fifth International Obsessive-Compulsive Disorder Conference, Sardinia, Italy, March 29-April 1, 2001

Hollander E, Koran LM, Goodman W, et al: A Double-blind, placebo-controlled study of the efficacy and safety of controlled release fluvoxamine in patients with obsessive-compulsive disorder. J Clin Psychiatry (in press, a)

Hollander E, Allen A, Steiner M, et al: Acute and long-term treatment and prevention of relapse in obsessive-complsive disorder with paroxetine. J Clin Psychiatry (in press, b)

Insel TR, Murphy DL, Cohen RM, et al: Obsessive-compulsive disorder: a double-blind trial of clomipramine and clorgyline. Arch Gen Psychiatry 40:605–612, 1983

The International Multicenter Clinical Trial Group on Moclobemide in Social Phobia: Moclobemide in social phobia: a double-blind, placebo-controlled study. Eur Arch Psychiatry Clin Neurosci 247:71–80, 1997

James IM, Griffith DNW, Pearson RM, et al: Effect of oxprenolol on stage-fright in musicians. Lancet 2:952–954, 1977

James IM, Borgoyne W, Savage IT: Effect of pindolol on stress-related disturbances of musical performance: preliminary communication. J R Soc Med 76:194–196, 1983

Jenike MA, Hyman S, Baer L, et al: A controlled trial of fluvoxamine in obsessive-compulsive disorder: implications for a serotonergic theory. Am J Psychiatry 147:1209–1215, 1990a

Jenike MA, Baer L, Summergrad P, et al: Sertraline in obsessive-compulsive disorder: a double-blind comparison with placebo. Am J Psychiatry 147:923–928, 1990b

Jenike MA, Baer L, Ballantine HT, et al: Cingulotomy for refractory obsessive-compulsive disorder: a long-term follow-up of 33 patients. Arch Gen Psychiatry 48:548–555, 1991

Jenike MA, Baer L, Minichiello WE, et al: Placebo-controlled trial of fluoxetine and phenelzine for obsessive-compulsive disorder. Am J Psychiatry 154:1261–1264, 1997

Kahn RJ, McNair DM, Lipman RS, et al: Imipramine and chlordiazepoxide in depressive and anxiety disorders, II: efficacy in anxious outpatients. Arch Gen Psychiatry 43:79–85, 1986

Katzelnick DJ, Kobak KA, Greist JH, et al: Sertraline for social phobia: a double-blind, placebo-controlled crossover study. Am J Psychiatry 152:1368–1371, 1995

Kauffman CD, Reist C, Djenderedjian A, et al: Biological markers of affective disorders and posttraumatic stress disorder: a pilot study with desipramine. J Clin Psychiatry 48:366–367, 1987

Keck PE, Taylor VE, Tugrul KC, et al: Valproate treatment of panic disorder and lactate-induced panic attacks. Biol Psychiatry 33:542–546, 1993

Kelsey JE: Venlafaxine in social phobia. Psychopharmacol Bull 31:767–771, 1995

Kinzie JD, Leung P: Clonidine in Cambodian patients with posttraumatic stress disorder. J Nerv Ment Dis 177:546–550, 1989

Klein DF: Delineation of two drug responsive anxiety syndromes. Psychopharmacologia 5:397–408, 1964

Kolb LC, Burris BC, Griffiths S: Propranolol and clonidine in treatment of the chronic post-traumatic stress disorders of war, in Post-Traumatic Stress Disorder: Psychological and Biological Sequelae. Edited by van der Kolk BA. Washington, DC, American Psychiatric Press, 1984, pp 97–105

Koran LM, McElroy SL, Davidson JR, et al: Fluvoxamine versus clomipramine for obsessive-compulsive disorder: a double-blind comparison. J Clin Psychopharmacol 16:121–129, 1996

Koran LM, Ringold AL, Elliott MA: Olanzapine augmentation for treatment-resistant obsessive-compulsive disorder. J Clin Psychiatry 61:514–517, 2000

Kronig MH, Apter J, Asnis G, et al: Placebo-controlled, multicenter study of sertraline treatment for obsessive-compulsive disorder. J Clin Psychopharmacol 19:172–176, 1999

Lecrubier Y, Judge R: Long-term evaluation of paroxetine, clomipramine and placebo in panic disorder. Collaborative Paroxetine Panic Study Investigators. Acta Psychiatr Scand 95:153–160, 1997

Lecrubier Y, Bakker A, Dunbar G, et al: A comparison of paroxetine, clomipramine and placebo in the treatment of panic disorder: Collaborative Paroxetine Panic Study Investigators. Acta Psychiatr Scand 95:145–152, 1997

Leonard HL, Swedo SE, Rapoport JL, et al: Treatment of obsessive-compulsive disorder with clomipramine and desipramine in children and adolescents: a double-blind crossover comparison. Arch Gen Psychiatry 46:1088–1092, 1989

Leonard HL, Swedo SE, Lenane MC, et al: A double-blind desipramine substitution during long-term clomipramine treatment in children and adolescents with obsessive-compulsive disorder. Arch Gen Psychiatry 48:922–927, 1991

Leonard HL, Swedo SE, Lenane MC, et al: A 2- to 7-year follow-up study of 54 obsessive compulsive children and adolescents. Arch Gen Psychiatry 50:429–439, 1993

Lepola UM, Wade AG, Leinonen EV, et al: A controlled, prospective, 1-year trial of citalopram in the treatment of panic disorder. J Clin Psychiatry 59:528–534, 1998

Liden S, Gottfries CG: Beta-blocking agents in the treatment of catecholamine-induced symptoms in musicians. Lancet 2:529, 1974

Liebowitz MR, Fyer AJ, McGrath P, et al: Clonidine treatment of panic disorder. Psychopharmcol Bull 17:122–123, 1981

Liebowitz MR, Schneier F, Campeas R, et al: Phenelzine vs atenolol in social phobia: a placebo-controlled comparison. Arch Gen Psychiatry 49:290–300, 1992

Lipper S, Davidson JRT, Grady TA, et al: Preliminary study of carbamazepine in post-traumatic stress disorder. Psychosomatics 27:849–854, 1986

Lippitz BE, Mindus P, Meyerson BA, et al: Lesion topography and outcome after thermocapsulotomy or gamma knife capsulotomy for obsessive-compulsive disorder: relevance of the right hemisphere. Neurosurgery 44:452–458, 1999

Londborg PD, Wolkow R, Smith WT, et al: Sertraline in the treatment of panic disorder: A multi-site, double-blind, placebo-controlled, fixed-dose investigation. Br J Psychiatry 173:54–60, 1998

Maletzky B, McFarland B, Burt A: Refractory obsessive compulsive disorder and ECT. Convuls Ther 10:34–42, 1994

March JS, Biederman J, Wolkow R, et al: Sertraline in children and adolescents with obsessive-compulsive disorder: a multicenter randomized controlled trial. JAMA 280:1752–1756, 1998

Marks IM, Stern RS, Mawson D, et al: Clomipramine and exposure for obsessive-compulsive rituals, I. Br J Psychiatry 136:1–25, 1980

Marshall JR: The treatment of night terrors associated with posttraumatic syndrome. Am J Psychiatry 132:293–295, 1975

Marshall RD, Schneier FR, Fallon BA, et al: An open trial of paroxetine in patients with noncombat-related, chronic posttraumatic stress disorder. J Clin Psychopharmacol 18:10–18, 1998

Mavissakalian M, Michelson L: Agoraphobia: relative and combined effectiveness of therapist-assisted in vivo exposure and imipramine. J Clin Psychiatry 47:117–122, 1986a

Mavissakalian M, Michelson L: Two-year follow-up of exposure and imipramine treatment of agoraphobia. Am J Psychiatry 143:1106–1112, 1986b

Mavissakalian M, Perel JM: Imipramine dose-response relationship in panic disorder with agoraphobia: preliminary findings. Arch Gen Psychiatry 46:127–131, 1989

Mavissakalian M, Perel JM: Clinical experiments in maintenance and discontinuation of imipramine therapy in panic disorder with agoraphobia. Arch Gen Psychiatry 49:318–323, 1992

Mavissakalian M, Perel JM: Imipramine treatment of panic disorder with agoraphobia: dose ranging and plasma level-response relationships. Am J Psychiatry 152:673–682, 1995

McCafferty JP, Bellew KM, Zaninelli RM: Paroxetine treatment of GAD: an analysis of response by dose. Paper presented at the annual meeting of the American Psychiatric Association, New Orleans, LA, May 2001

McDougle CJ, Goodman WK, Price LH, et al: Neuroleptic addition in fluvoxamine-refractory obsessive-compulsive disorder. Am J Psychiatry 147:652–654, 1990

McDougle CJ, Price LH, Goodman WK, et al: A controlled trial of lithium augmentation in fluvoxamine-refractory obsessive-compulsive disorder: lack of efficacy. J Clin Psychopharmacol 11:175–181, 1991a

McDougle CJ, Southwick SM, Charney DS, et al: An open trial of fluoxetine in the treatment of posttraumatic stress disorder. J Clin Psychopharmacol 11:325–327, 1991b

McDougle CJ, Goodman WK, Leckman JF, et al: The efficacy of fluvoxamine in obsessive-compulsive disorder: effects of comorbid chronic tic disorder. J Clin Psychopharmacol 13:354–358, 1993a

McDougle CJ, Goodman WK, Leckman JF, et al: Limited therapeutic effect of addition of buspirone in fluvoxamine-refractory obsessive-compulsive disorder. Am J Psychiatry 150:647–649, 1993b

McDougle CJ, Goodman WK, Leckman JF, et al: Haloperidol addition in fluvoxamine-refractory obsessive-compulsive disorder. A double-blind, placebo-controlled study in patients with and without tics. Arch Gen Psychiatry 51:302–308, 1994

McDougle CJ, Epperson CN, Pelton GH, et al: A double-blind, placebo-controlled study of risperidone addition in serotonin reuptake inhibitor-refractory obsessive-compulsive disorder. Arch Gen Psychiatry 57:794–801, 2000

McNair DM, Kahn RJ: Imipramine compared with a benzodiazepine for agoraphobia, in Anxiety: New Research and Changing Concepts. Edited by Klein DF, Rabkin JG. New York, Raven, 1981, pp 69–80

Michelson D, Lydiard RB, Pollack MH, et al: Outcome assessment and clinical improvement in panic disorder: evidence from a randomized controlled trial of fluoxetine and placebo: The Fluoxetine Panic Disorder Study Group. Am J Psychiatry 155:1570–1577, 1998

Michelson D, Pollack M, Lydiard RB, et al: Continuing treatment of panic disorder after acute response: randomized, placebo-controlled trial with fluoxetine: The Fluoxetine Panic Disorder Study Group. Br J Psychiatry 174:213–218, 1999

Mindus, Jenike MA: Neurosurgical treatment of malignant obsessive-compulsive disorder. Psychiatr Clin North Am 15:921–938, 1992

Montgomery SA, McIntyre A, Osterheider M, et al: A double-blind, placebo-controlled study of fluoxetine in patients with DSM-III-R obsessive-compulsive disorder. The Lilly European OCD Study Group. Eur Neuropsychopharmacol 3:143–152, 1993

Mountjoy CQ, Roth M, Garside RF, et al: A clinical trial of phenelzine in anxiety depressive and phobic neuroses. Br J Psychiatry 131:486–492, 1977

Mundo E, Richter MA, Sam F, et al: Is the 5-HT(1Dbeta) receptor gene implicated in the pathogenesis of obsessive-compulsive disorder? Am J Psychiatry 157:1160–1161, 2000

Nagy LM, Krystal JH, Woods SW, et al: Clinical and medication outcome after short-term alprazolam and behavioral group treatment in panic disorder: 2.5-year naturalistic follow-up study. Arch Gen Psychiatry 46:993–999, 1989

Neftel KA, Adler RH, Kappell K, et al: Stage fright in musicians: a model illustrating the effect of beta blockers. Psychosom Med 44:461–469, 1982

Nicolson R, Swedo SE, Lenane M, et al: An open trial of plasma exchange in childhood-onset obsessive-compulsive disorder without posttreptococcal exacerbations. J Am Acad Child Adolesc Psychiatry 39:1313–1315, 2000

Noyes R Jr, Garvey MJ, Cook BL: Follow-up study of patients with panic disorder and agoraphobia with panic attacks treated with tricyclic antidepressants. J Affect Disord 16:249–257, 1989

Noyes R Jr, Moroz G, Davidson JRT, et al: Moclobemide in social phobia: a controlled dose-response trial. J Clin Psychopharmacol 17:247–254, 1997

Oehrberg S, Christiansen PE, Behnke K, et al: Paroxetine in the treatment of panic disorder. A randomized, double-blind, placebo-controlled study. Br J Psychiatry 167:374–379, 1995

Otto MW, Pollack MH, Sachs GS, et al: Discontinuation of benzodiazepine treatment: efficacy of cognitive-behavioral therapy for patients with panic disorder. Am J Psychiatry 150:1485–1490, 1993

Pallanti S, Quercioli L, Paiva RS, et al: Citalopram for treatment-resistant obsessive-compulsive disorder. Eur Psychiatry 14:101–106, 1999

Pande AC, Davidson JRT, Jefferson JW, et al: Treatment of social phobia with gabapentin: a placebo-controlled study. J Clin Psychopharmacol 19:341–348, 1999

Pande AC, Pollack MH, Crockattt J, et al: Placebo-controlled study of gabapentin treatment of panic disorder. J Clin Psychopharmacol 20:467–471, 2000

Papp LA, Coplan JD, Marinez JM, et al: Efficacy of open-label nefazodone treatment in patients with panic disorder. J Clin Psychopharmacol 20:544–546, 2000

Pato MT, Zohar-Kadouch R, Zohar J, et al: Return of symptoms after discontinuation of clomipramine in patients with obsessive-compulsive disorder. Am J Psychiatry 145:1521–1525, 1988

Pato MT, Pigott TA, Hill JL, et al: Controlled comparison of buspirone and clomipramine in obsessive-compulsive disorder. Am J Psychiatry 148:127–129, 1991

Pecknold JC, Swinson RP, Kuch K, et al: Alprazolam in panic disorder and agoraphobia: results from a multicenter trial, III: discontinuation effects. Arch Gen Psychiatry 45:429–436, 1988

Perlmutter SJ, Leitman SF, Garvey MA, et al: Therapeutic plasma exchange and intravenous immunoglobulin for obsessive-compulsive disorder and tic disorders in childhood. Lancet 354:1153–1158, 1999

Perse TL, Greist JH, Jefferson JW, et al: Fluvoxamine treatment of obsessive-compulsive disorder. Am J Psychiatry 144:1543–1548, 1987

Pfanner C, Marazziti D, Dell'Osso L, et al: Risperidone augmentation in refractory obsessive-compulsive disorder: an open-label study. Int Clin Psychopharmacol 15:297–301, 2000

Piccinelli M, Pini S, Bellantuono C, et al: Efficacy of drug treatment in obsessive-compulsive disorder. A meta-analytic review. Br J Psychiatry 166:424–443, 1995

Pigott TA, Pato MT, Bernstein SE, et al: Controlled comparisons of clomipramine and fluoxetine in the treatment of obsessive-compulsive disorder: behavioral and biological results. Arch Gen Psychiatry 47:926–932, 1990

Pigott TA, Pato MT, L'Heureux F, et al: A controlled comparison of adjuvant lithium carbonate or thyroid hormone in clomipramine-treated patients with obsessive-compulsive disorder. J Clin Psychopharmacol 11:242–248, 1991

Pigott TA, L'Heureux F, Hill JL, et al: A double-blind study of adjuvant buspirone hydrochloride in clomipramine-treated patients with obsessive-compulsive disorder. J Clin Psychopharmacol 12:11–18, 1992a

Pigott TA, L'Heureux F, Rubenstein CS, et al: A double-blind, placebo controlled study of trazodone in patients with obsessive-compulsive disorder. J Clin Psychopharmacol 12:156–162, 1992b

Pohl RB, Wolkow RM, Clary CM: Sertraline in the treatment of panic disorder: a double-blind multicenter trial. Am J Psychiatry 155:1189–1195, 1998

Pollack MH, Worthington JJ 3rd, Otto MW, et al: Venlafaxine for panic disorder: results of a double-blind, placebo-controlled study. Psychopharmacol Bull 32:667–670, 1996

Pollack MH, Zaninelli R, Goddard A, et al: Paroxetine in the treatment of generalized anxiety disorder: results of a placebo-controlled, flexible-dosage trial. J Clin Psychiatry 62:350–357, 2001

Rapaport MH, Pollack MH, Clary CM, et al: Panic disorder and response to sertraline: the effect of previous treatment with benzodiazepines. J Clin Psychopharmacol 21:104–107, 2001

Raskind MA, Thompson C, Petrie EC, et al: Prazosin reduces nightmares in combat veterans with posttraumatic stress disorder. J Clin Psychiatry 63(7):565–568, 2002

Rasmussen S, Hackett E, DuBoff E, et al: A 2-year study of sertraline in the treatment of obsessive-compulsive disorder. Int Clin Psychopharmacol 12:309–316, 1997

Ravizza L, Barzega G, Bellino S, et al: Predictors of drug treatment response in obsessive-compulsive disorder. J Clin Psychiatry 56:368–373, 1995

Ravizza L, Albert U, Ceregato A: Venlafaxine in OCD. Presented at the Fifth International Obsessive-Compulsive Disorder Conference, Sardinia, Italy, March 29-April 1, 2001

Reist C, Kauffmann CD, Haier RJ, et al: A controlled trial of desipramine in 18 men with posttraumatic stress disorder. Am J Psychiatry 146:513–516, 1989

Rickels K, Csanalosi I, Greisman P, et al: A controlled clinical trial of alprazolam for the treatment of anxiety. Am J Psychiatry 140:82–85, 1983

Rickels K, Schweizer E, Csanalosi I, et al: Long-term treatment of anxiety and risk of withdrawal: prospective comparison of clorazepate and buspirone. Arch Gen Psychiatry 45:444–450, 1988

Rickels K, Schweizer E, Weiss S, et al: Maintenance drug treatment for panic disorder, II: short- and long-term outcome after drug taper. Arch Gen Psychiatry 50:61–68, 1993a

Rickels K, Downing R, Schweizer E, et al: Antidepressants for the treatment of generalized anxiety disorder. A placebo-controlled comparison of imipramine, trazodone, and diazepam. Arch Gen Psychiatry 50:884–895, 1993b

Rickels K, DeMartinis N, Garcia-Espana F, et al: Imipramine and buspirone in treatment of patients with generalized anxiety disorder who are discontinuing long-term benzodiazepine therapy. Am J Psychiatry 157:1973–1979, 2000a

Rickels K, Pollack MH, Sheehan DV, et al: Efficacy of extended-release venlafaxine in nondepressed outpatients with generalized anxiety disorder. Am J Psychiatry 157:968–974, 2000b

Riddle MA, Scahill L, King RA, et al: Double-blind, crossover trial of fluoxetine and placebo in children and adolescents with obsessive-compulsive disorder. J Am Acad Child Adolesc Psychiatry 31:1062–1069, 1992

Riddle MA, Reeve EA, Yaryura-Tobias JA, et al: Fluvoxamine for children and adolescents with obsessive-compulsive disorder: a randomized, controlled, multicenter trial. J Am Acad Child Adolesc Psychiatry 40:222–229, 2001

Rocca P, Fonzo V, Scotta M, et al: Paroxetine efficacy in the treatment of generalized anxiety disorder. Acta Psychiatr Scand 95:444–450, 1997

Romach M, Busto U, Somer G, et al: Clinical aspects of chronic use of alprazolam and lorazepam. Am J Psychiatry 152:1161–1167, 1995

Romano S, Goodman W, Tamura R, et al: Long-term treatment of obsessive-compulsive disorder after an acute response: a comparison of fluoxetine versus placebo. J Clin Psychopharmacol 21:46–52, 2001

Rosenberg DR, Stewart CM, Fitzgerald KD, et al: Paroxetine open-label treatment of pediatric outpatients with obsessive-compulsive disorder. J Am Acad Child Adolesc Psychiatry 38:1180–1185, 1999

Rosenbaum JF, Moroz G, Bowden CL: Clonazepam in the treatment of panic disorder with or without agoraphobia: a dose-response study of efficacy, safety, and discontinuance: Clonazepam Panic Disorder Dose-Response Study Group. J Clin Psychopharmacol 17:390–400, 1997

Ruiz AT: A double-blind study of alprazolam and lorazepam in the treatment of anxiety. J Clin Psychiatry 44:60–62, 1983

Saxena S, Wang D, Bystritsky A, et al: Risperidone augmentation of SRI treatment for refractory obsessive-compulsive disorder. J Clin Psychiatry 57:303–306, 1996

Schneier FR, Saoud JB, Campeas R, et al: Buspirone in social phobia. J Clin Psychopharmacol 13:251–256, 1993

Schneier FR, Goetz D, Campeas R, et al: Placebo-controlled trial of moclobemide in social phobia. Br J Psychiatry 172:70–77, 1998

Schweizer E, Rickels K, Lucki I: Resistance to the anti-anxiety effect of buspirone in patients with a history of benzodiazepine use. N Engl J Med 314:719–720, 1986

Schweizer E, Rickels K, Weiss S, et al: Maintenance drug treatment of panic disorder. I. Results of a prospective, placebo-controlled comparison of alprazolam and imipramine. Arch Gen Psychiatry 50:51–60, 1993

Seedat S, Stein DJ: Inositol augmentation of serotonin reuptake inhibitors in treatment-refractory obsessive-compulsive disorder: an open trial. Int Clin Psychopharmacol 14:353–356, 1999

Seedat S, Stein JD, Emsley RA: Open trial of citalopram in adults with posttraumatic stress disorder. Int J Neuropsychopharmacol 3:135–140, 2000

Seedat S, Lockhart R, Kaminer D, et al: An open trial of citalopram in adolescents with post-traumatic stress disorder. Int Clin Psychopharmacol 16:21–25, 2001

Sheehan DV, Ballenger J, Jacobsen G: Treatment of endogenous anxiety with phobic, hysterical, and hypochondriacal symptoms. Arch Gen Psychiatry 37:51–59, 1980

Solyom L, Heseltine GFD, McClure DJ, et al: Behavior therapy versus drug therapy in the treatment of phobic neurosis. Can J Psychiatry 18:25–32, 1973

Solyom C, Solyom K, LaPierre Y, et al: Phenelzine and exposure in the treatment of phobias. Biol Psychiatry 16:239–247, 1981

Spiegel DA, Bruce TJ, Gregg SF, et al: Does cognitive behavior therapy assist slow-taper alprazolam discontinuation in panic disorder? Am J Psychiatry 151:876–881, 1994

Stein DJ, Spadaccine E, Hollander E: Meta-analysis of pharmacotherapy trials for obsessive-compulsive disorder. Int Clin Psychopharmacol 10:11–18, 1995

Stein MB, Liebowitz MR, Lydiard B, et al: Paroxetine treatment of generalized social phobia (social anxiety disorder): a randomized controlled trial. JAMA 280:708–713, 1998

Stein MB, Fyer AJ, Davidson JRT, et al: Fluvoxamine treatment of social phobia (social anxiety disorder): a double-blind, placebo-controlled study. Am J Psychiatry 156:756–760, 1999

Szegedi A, Wetzel H, Leal M, et al: Combination treatment with clomipramine and fluvoxamine: drug monitoring, safety, and tolerability data. J Clin Psychiatry 57:257–264, 1996

Szymanski HV, Olympia J: Divalproex in posttraumatic stress disorder (letter). Am J Psychiatry 148:1086–1087, 1991

Thomsen PH: Child and adolescent obsessive-compulsive disorder treated with citalopram: findings from an open trial of 23 cases. J Child Adolesc Psychopharmacol 7:157–166, 1997

Thorén P, Åsberg M, Cronholm B, et al: Clomipramine treatment of obsessive-compulsive disorder, I: a controlled clinical trial. Arch Gen Psychiatry 37:1281–1285, 1980.

Tiffon L, Coplan JD, Papp LA et al: Augmentation strategies with tricyclic or fluoxetine treatment in seven partially responsive panic disorder patients. J Clin Psychiatry 55:66–69, 1994

Tollefson GD, Rampey AH, Potvin JH, et al: A multicenter investigation of fixed-dose fluoxetine in the treatment of obsessive-compulsive disorder. Arch Gen Psychiatry 51:559–567, 1994

Tyrer P, Candy J, Kelly D: A study of the clinical effects of phenelzine and placebo in the treatment of phobic anxiety. Psychopharmacology (Berl) 32:237–254, 1973

Uhde TW, Stein MB, Vittone BJ, et al: Behavioral and physiologic effects of short-term and long-term administration of clonidine in panic disorder. Arch Gen Psychiatry 46:170–177, 1989

Vallejo J, Olivares J, Marcos T, et al: Clomipramine versus phenelzine in obsessive-compulsive disorder: a controlled clinical trial. Br J Psychiatry 161:665–670, 1992

Van Ameringen M, Mancini C, Streiner DL: Fluoxetine efficacy in social phobia. J Clin Psychiatry 54:27–32, 1993

Van Ameringen M, Mancini C, Streiner D: Sertraline in social phobia. J Affect Disord 31:141–145, 1994

Van Ameringen M, Mancini C, Oakman JM: Nefazodone in social phobia. J Clin Psychiatry 60:96–100, 1999

Van Ameringen MA, Lane RM, Walker JR, et al: Sertraline treatment of generalized social phobia: a 20-week, double-blind, placebo-controlled study. Am J Psychiatry 158:275–281, 2001

van der Kolk BA: Psychopharmacological issues in posttraumatic stress disorder. Hosp Community Psychiatry 34:683–691, 1983

van der Kolk BA, Dreyfuss D, Michaels M, et al: Fluoxetine in posttraumatic stress disorder. J Clin Psychiatry 55:517–522, 1994

van Vliet IM, den Boer JA, Westenberg HG: Psychopharmacological treatment of social phobia; a double blind placebo controlled study with fluvoxamine. Psychopharmacology (Berl) 115:128–134, 1994

van Vliet IM, den Boer JA, Westenberg HGM, et al: Clinical effects of buspirone in social phobia: a double-blind placebo-controlled study. J Clin Psychiatry 58:164–168, 1997

Versiani M, Mundim FD, Nardi AE, et al: Tranylcypromine in social phobia. J Clin Psychopharmacol 8:279–283, 1988

Wade AG, Lepola U, Koponen HJ, et al: The effect of citalopram in panic disorder. Br J Psychiatry 170:549–553, 1997

Warneke LB: Intravenous chlorimipramine in the treatment of obsessional disorder in adolescence: case report. J Clin Psychiatry 46:100–103, 1985

Weiss EL, Potenza MN, McDougle CJ, et al: Olanzapinen addition in obsessive-compulsive disorder refractory to selective serotonin reuptake inhibitors: an open-label case series. J Clin Psychiatry 60:524–527, 1999

Wolf ME, Alavi A, Mosnaim AD: Posttraumatic stress disorder in Vietnam veterans, clinical and EEG findings: possible therapeutic effects of carbamazepine. Biol Psychiatry 23:642–644, 1988

Woodman CL, Noyes R: Panic disorder: treatment with valproate. J Clin Psychiatry 55:134–136, 1994

Zisook S, Chentsova-Dutton YE, Smith-Vaniz A, et al: Nefazodone in patients with treatment-refractory posttraumatic stress disorder. J Clin Psychiatry 61:203–208, 2000

Zitrin CM, Klein DF, Woerner MG: Treatment of agoraphobia with group exposure in vivo and imipramine. Arch Gen Psychiatry 37:63–72, 1980

Zitrin CM, Klein DF, Woerner MG, et al: Treatment of phobias, I: comparison of imipramine hydrochloride and placebo. Arch Gen Psychiatry 40:125–138, 1983

Zohar J, Insel TR: Obsessive-compulsive disorder: psychobiological approaches to diagnosis, treatment, and pathophysiology. Biol Psychiatry 22:667–687, 1987

7

PSYCHOTHERAPY
TREATMENTS

■ PANIC DISORDER

Psychodynamic Psychotherapy

Even after medication has blocked the actual panic attacks, a sub-group of patients with panic disorder remains wary of independence and assertiveness. In addition to supportive and behavioral treatment, traditional psychodynamic psychotherapy might be helpful for some of these patients. Significant unconscious conflict over separations during childhood sometimes appears to operate in patients with panic disorder, leading to a reemergence of anxiety symptoms in adult life each time a new separation is imagined or threatened. Furthermore, it has been found that comorbid personality disorder is the major predictor of continued social maladjustment in patients otherwise treated for panic disorder (Noyes et al. 1990), suggesting that psychodynamic therapy may be an important additional treatment for at least some patients with panic disorder.

Unfortunately, there are few systematic studies documenting the efficacy of psychodynamic psychotherapy in panic disorder. Clinicians with a psychodynamic orientation tend to agree that psychological factors do not appear to be prominent in many patients with panic disorder and emphasize the importance of conducting a psychodynamic assessment to determine whether a particular patient may or may not benefit from a psychodynamic treatment component (Gabbard 1990). Moreover, Cooper (1985) has emphasized that in those patients with a predominant biological component to their illness, insistence on dynamic understanding and on responsibility for one's symptoms may be, in the long run, not only useless but potentially harmful, leading to further damage in self-esteem and strengthened masochistic defenses. However, it is also clear that there are case reports of patients who were successfully treated for panic with psychodynamic therapy or psychoanalysis.

A recent controlled study showed that a 15-session course of brief dynamic psychotherapy combined with initial medication (clomipramine) treatment led to much lower relapse rates up to 9 months after the medication had been tapered off (Wiborg and Dahl 1996). More recently, an open trial of psychodynamic monotherapy in panic disorder documented clear efficacy for this modality, at least in the selected sample, and emphasizes the need for further and controlled studies (Milrod et al. 2000). The study included 14 patients with panic disorder who were treated for 12 weeks with twice-weekly psychodynamic psychotherapy alone; the patients showed notable improvement in panic, anxiety, depression, and overall impairment at the end of the 12 weeks and at 6-month follow-up.

Pharmacotherapy is in no way incompatible with behavioral or psychodynamic treatment for patients with panic disorder. The notion that reducing the symptoms of anxiety disorder with medication will disturb a successful psychotherapy is outdated and largely dogmatic. Indeed, it is often true that successful psychotherapy cannot take place until the more debilitating aspects of these syndromes have been eliminated pharmacologically.

Supportive Psychotherapy

Despite adequate treatment of panic attacks with medication, phobic avoidance can still remain, and supportive psychotherapy and education about the illness are necessary to urge the patient to confront the phobic situation. Patients for whom supportive interventions are not effective may then need additional psychotherapy—dynamic or cognitive-behavioral. Encouragement from other patients with similar conditions is often quite helpful, and group treatment can be very useful in this regard.

Cognitive and Behavioral Therapy

In recent years, interest in cognitive and behavioral therapy for panic disorder has surged, and cognitive and behavioral therapies have become firmly established as first-line treatment options for this disorder. Treatments had long focused on phobic avoidance, but more recently, effective techniques have been developed and shown to be effective for panic attacks per se. With regard to the agoraphobic component that can be present in panic disorder, it has been long established that situational exposure is the most effective treatment (Agras et al. 1968). This treatment involves teaching patients to gradually expose themselves to real-life situations that they have been avoiding, starting with the least anxiety provoking situations and progressing to situations that are more and more challenging. This gradual systematic exposure leads to marked improvement of phobic avoidance in most patients, although usually treatment of the panic attacks must also be addressed in order to achieve maximal results.

The major behavioral techniques for the treatment of the panic attacks per se are breathing retraining to control both acute and chronic hyperventilation; exposure to somatic cues, usually involving a hierarchy of exposure to feared sensations through imaginal and behavioral exercises; and relaxation training. The comprehensive treatment packet for panic disorder that was developed by Barlow and colleagues is primarily behavioral and is referred to as *panic control treatment* (Barlow et al. 1989). It combines interoceptive exposure to treat the attacks, situational exposure to treat the avoidance, and elements of education and cognitive restructuring. In the original controlled study of panic control treatment, more than 80% of study participants treated solely with panic control treatment were free of panic after 12 weeks of sessions, and the addition of a muscle relaxation component appeared to add very little to the success of the treatment; relaxation alone was not significantly better than the waiting-list placebo control condition (Barlow et al. 1989). Remarkably, more than 80% of the study participants who had received panic control treatment remained free of panic at 2-year follow-up; again, relaxation alone or as a supplement to the panic control treatment did not appear to be helpful and may even have been detrimental (Craske et al. 1991). This panic control treatment has also been successfully applied in a group format with similar findings: again more than 80% of patients becoming panic-free after 8 weeks of sessions (Telch et al. 1993).

The cognitive treatment of panic attacks centers on more intensive cognitive restructuring, which allows the patient to learn a more benign interpretation, with less sense of catastrophe, to the uncomfortable affects and physical sensations associated with the attacks (Beck et al. 1985; Clark 1988). These cognitive techniques can be administered in various combinations and appear to be overall quite effective in treating the disorder (Salkovskis 1986; Sokol et al. 1989). In one study, more than 70% of patients treated for 8 weeks with focused cognitive therapy for panic disorder became panic free, compared with 25% in the supportive therapy group. At 1-year follow-up, almost 90% of the patients who had received cognitive therapy remained free of panic (Beck et al. 1992). The extreme cognitive view is that panic attacks consist of normal physical sensations (e.g., palpitations, slight dizziness) to which panic disorder patients grossly overreact with catastrophic cognitions. A more middle-of-the-road view is that panic disorder patients do have extreme physical sensations such as bursts of tachycardia but can still help themselves greatly by changing their interpretation of the event from "I am going to die of a heart attack!" to "There go my heart symptoms again." This benign cognitive restructuring acts to block the further escalation of physical symptoms, referred to as *the fear of fear* (Goldstein and Chambless 1978), into full-blown attacks. Such a model has received experimental validation: Sanderson and colleagues (1989) provoked panic attacks in panic disorder patients with carbon dioxide inhalation; it was found that when patients had an illusion of control over the inhaled mixture, they experienced notably fewer and less severe attacks and had less catastrophic cognitions. Findings have been somewhat inconsistent as to whether applied relaxation is equally efficacious or inferior to cognitive-behavioral therapy (CBT) in controlling panic attacks (Arntz and van den Hout 1996Ost and Westling 1995;).

Cognitive and behavioral approaches to the treatment of panic disorder are summarized in Table 7–1. In effect, elements of both approaches are commonly combined for optimal outcome.

■ GENERALIZED ANXIETY DISORDER

Research into the psychotherapy of generalized anxiety disorder (GAD) has not been as extensive as for other anxiety disorders. Still, a number of studies exist that clearly show that a variety of psychotherapies are helpful in treating GAD. Cognitive and behavioral approaches to treating GAD are listed in Table 7–2. Given the previously described cognitive profile of GAD (see Chapter 5, "Psychological Theories"), several aspects of the disorder can serve as the foci of psychotherapeutic interventions. These include the heightened tendency to perceive threat; the expectation of low-likelihood catastrophic outcomes; poor problem solving, especially in the face of ambivalence or ambiguity; the central feature, worry; and the physical symptoms of anxiety. A variety of treatments have been developed for GAD, including cognitive restructuring; behavioral anxiety management, such as relaxation and breathing techniques; exposure therapy, with or without a cognitive component; and psychodynamic treatment.

TABLE 7–1. **Cognitive and behavioral approaches to treating panic disorder**

Interoceptive exposure (to the somatic cues of panic attacks)
Situational exposure (to the settings that are phobically avoided)
Cognitive restructuring
Breathing retraining
Applied relaxation training

TABLE 7–2.	Cognitive and behavioral approaches to treating generalized anxiety disorder

Exposure
Cognitive restructuring
Breathing retraining
Applied relaxation training

CBT is superior to general nondirective or supportive therapy in treating GAD (Chambless and Gillis 1993), and possibly superior to behavioral therapy alone (Borkovec and Costello 1993). Cognitive therapy alone may have an edge over behavioral therapy alone, according to some studies (Butler et al. 1991) but not others (Ost and Breitholtz 2000). In a study that compared four conditions, behavioral therapy alone, cognitive therapy alone, CBT, and a waiting list control group, all three active treatments were similarly efficacious and superior to the control condition during a follow-up period of up to 2 years. However, the combined CBT group had a much lower dropout rate than the other groups (Barlow et al. 1992). Another randomized study compared cognitive, analytic, and behavioral management in treating patients with GAD (Durham et al. 1994). Cognitive therapy emerged as superior, with a slight advantage over behavioral management alone and significantly better than analytic treatment. Biofeedback is an additional treatment that may have some efficacy in treating GAD (Rice et al. 1993).

■ SOCIAL PHOBIA

Cognitive and Behavioral Therapy

Three major cognitive-behavioral techniques are used very effectively in the treatment of social phobia: exposure, cognitive restructuring, and social skills training (Table 7–3). Exposure treatment involves imaginal or in vivo exposure to specific feared performance and social situations. Although patients with very high lev-

TABLE 7–3.	**Cognitive and behavioral approaches to treating social phobia**

Cognitive restructuring
Exposure (imaginal and/or in vivo)
Social skills training (modeling, rehearsal, role-playing, practice)

els of social anxiety may need to begin with imaginal exposure until a certain degree of habituation is attained, therapeutic results are not gained until in vivo exposure is carried out in the real-life feared situations. Social skills training employs modeling, rehearsal, role playing, and assigned practice to help persons learn appropriate behaviors and decrease their anxiety in social situations, with an expectation that accomplishment will lead to more positive responses from others. This type of training is not necessary for all persons with social phobia; it is more applicable to those who have actual deficits in social interacting above and beyond their anxiety or avoidance of social situations. Cognitive restructuring focuses on poor self-concepts, the fear of negative evaluation by others, and the attribution of positive outcomes to chance or circumstance and negative outcomes to one's own shortcomings. Cognitive restructuring consists of a variety of homework assignments: identifying negative thoughts, evaluating their accuracy, and reframing them in a more realistic way.

Results of older studies of behavioral treatments for social phobia were difficult to evaluate because of heterogeneous samples of patients with phobia, lack of operational definitions of disorder and improvement ratings, and the presentation of outcome data in terms of mean change scores rather than level of achieved functioning. However, in the past decade or so, CBT for social phobia has blossomed and attracted great attention, detailed treatment strategies and approaches have been delineated, and more thorough systematic studies in well-defined clinical populations have emerged.

Recent studies show that exposure, cognitive restructuring, and social skills training may all be of significant benefit to patients with social phobia. In addition, these techniques appear superior to non-specific supportive therapy, as shown in a randomized controlled study comparing supportive therapy to initial individual CBT followed by group social skills training (Cottraux et al. 2000). The success of CBT appears to be mediated, at least in part, by a decrease in self-focused attention (Woody et al. 1997). Attempts to correlate symptoms (e.g., social skills deficits, phobic anxiety, avoidance) with their proven treatments (social skills training, exposure) have not always been fruitful (Wlazlo et al. 1990). Heimberg and colleagues (1990) compared group CBT to a credible educational-supportive control intervention in patients with DSM-III (American Psychiatric Association 1980) social phobia; patients in both groups got better, but the CBT group showed more improvement, especially according to patients' self-appraisal. Finally, it has been suggested that cognitive factors may be of greater importance in social phobia than in other anxiety or phobic conditions, and therefore cognitive restructuring may be a necessary component to maximize treatment gains. Mattick and colleagues (1989) reported that combination treatment was superior to either exposure or cognitive restructuring alone in social phobia; cognitive restructuring alone was inferior to exposure alone in decreasing avoidant behavior, but exposure alone did not change self-perception and attitude.

Although long-term outcome is more difficult to assess, studies suggest that CBT leads to long-lasting gains (Turner et al. 1995) and therefore may be of particular significance in this disorder, which tends to have a chronic, often lifelong, course. At this point, it appears that in vivo exposure is a critical component of the treatment, and that the introduction of cognitive restructuring at some point in the treatment contributes to further gains and to their long-term maintenance. Social phobia is a disorder that often starts in the early years, and it is encouraging to know that for prepubertal children, both behavioral therapy—consisting of social skills training and anxiety reduction techniques (Beidel et al. 2000)—and CBT, alone or with the parents (Spence et al. 2000), have been found to be highly effective in controlled trials.

Other Psychotherapy

In recent years, the successful use of medication and behavioral treatments has resulted in psychodynamic therapy for phobias falling out of favor to some degree (Gabbard 1990). However, for those patients in whom underlying conflicts associated with phobic anxiety and avoidance can be identified by the clinician and that lend themselves to insightful exploration, psychodynamic therapy may be of benefit. One goal of psychodynamic therapy would be to uncover and work through either the oedipal conflicts that may undermine the patient's capacity for social success, or the disturbed object relationships involving harsh, critical introjects or identifications with others with social phobia that may underlie the patient's social phobia. Furthermore, a psychodynamic approach may be valuable in understanding and resolving the secondary interpersonal ramifications in which phobia patients and their partners are often caught that can operate as resistances to the successful implementation of medication or behavioral treatments (Gabbard 1990). In a recent trial of interpersonal psychotherapy adapted to treating social phobia, seven of nine patients treated openly for 14 weeks showed notable improvement (Lipsitz et al. 1999)—suggesting that this modality also merits further study.

■ SPECIFIC PHOBIA: BEHAVIORAL THERAPY

The behavioral therapy widely used for specific phobia is exposure. The problem lies in persuading the patient that exposure is worth trying and will be beneficial. Exposure treatments may be divided into two groups depending on whether exposure to the phobic object is *in vivo* or *imaginal*. In vivo exposure involves the patient in real-life contact with the phobic stimulus. Imaginal techniques confront the phobic stimulus through the therapist's descriptions and the patient's imagination.

The method of exposure in both the in vivo and imaginal techniques can be graded or ungraded. Graded exposure uses a hierarchy of anxiety-provoking events, varying from least to most stressful. The patient begins at the least stressful level and gradually progresses up the hierarchy. Ungraded exposure begins with the patient's confronting the most stressful items in the hierarchy.

Most exposure techniques have been used in both individual and group settings. (In a group setting, the example and the encouragement of other members are often particularly helpful in persuading the patient to reenter the phobic situation.) Exposure techniques include systematic desensitization, imaginal flooding, prolonged in vivo exposure, behavioral modeling, and reinforced practice.

Studies thus far have not conclusively shown any one exposure technique to be superior to other techniques or to be specifically indicated for particular phobia subtypes. In those patients whose phobic symptoms include panic attacks, antipanic medication may also be indicated.

■ OBSESSIVE-COMPULSIVE DISORDER

Behavioral Therapy

Behavioral treatments of obsessive-compulsive disorder (OCD) involve two separate components: 1) exposure procedures that aim to decrease the anxiety associated with obsessions or facing obsessional fears, and 2) response prevention techniques that aim to decrease the frequency of rituals or obsessive thoughts. Exposure techniques range from systematic desensitization with brief imaginal exposure, to flooding, in which prolonged exposure to the real-life ritual-evoking stimuli causes profound discomfort. Exposure techniques aim to ultimately decrease the discomfort associated with the eliciting stimuli through habituation. In exposure therapy, the patient is assigned homework exercises that must be adhered to, and the patient may require assistance in achieving exposure at home via the therapist's home visits or from family members. Response prevention involves having patients face feared stimuli (e.g., dirt, chemicals) without excessive hand washing, or tolerating doubt (e.g., "Is the door really locked?") without excessive checking. Initial work may involve delaying performance of the ritual, but ultimately the patient works to fully resist the compulsions. The education and support of family members is pivotal to the success of the behavioral therapy, because family dysfunction is very prevalent and the majority of parents or spouses accommodate to or are involved in the patients' rituals, possibly as a way to reduce the anxiety or anger that patients may direct at their family members (Calvocoressi et al. 1995; Shafran et al. 1996).

It is generally agreed that combined behavioral techniques (i.e., exposure with response prevention) yield the greatest improvement. It is also generally reported that patients who primarily have obsessions and have few rituals are the least responsive to behavioral treatment, although some behavioral techniques for obsessions may be promising (Salkovskis and Westbrook 1989). Using the combined techniques of in vivo exposure and response prevention, up to 75% of ritualizing patients willing and able to undergo the arduous treatment were reported to show significant improvement (Marks et al. 1975). The addition of imaginal exposure to in vivo exposure and response prevention is reported to help maintain treatment gains, perhaps by moderating obsessive fears of future catastrophes (Steketee et al. 1982). Foa and her group (Foa et al. 1984) systematically compared in vivo exposure, response prevention, and the two treatments combined. Patients in each of the treatment groups improved, but the combined treatment was superior in decreasing anxiety, rituals, and overall impairment. Clinical responders (defined as those patients who showed at least 30% improvement with treatment) comprised the following: 33% of the patients in the response-prevention group, 55% of those treated by exposure alone, and 90% of those who received combination treatment. It is interesting that this same study found that the majority of OCD patients successfully treated with behavioral therapy had relapsed at follow-up, suggesting that, just as with medication, long-term behavioral maintenance treatment may be necessary. Predictors of poorer outcome for behavioral treatment of OCD include initial depression, initial OCD severity, longer duration of the disorder, and lower motivation for treatment (Keijsers et al. 1994). Exposure and response prevention has also been used successfully to treat children and adolescents with OCD, and at least 50% improvement in the vast majority of study subjects has been reported (Franklin et al. 1998). A maintenance program can be highly effective in helping patients maintain their benefits from CBT over several years of follow-up (Marks 1997; McKay 1997). Also of interest is the question of the degree to which the results of controlled behavioral therapy trials—in which highly selected individuals are enrolled—generalize to broader community samples. A recent study investigated this important question and found comparable success in exposure and response prevention therapy carried out in an outpatient fee-for-service setting (Franklin et al. 2000).

It is not yet well known how behavioral techniques compare with medications in treating OCD. Marks and colleagues reported that self-managed exposure constitutes the most powerful treatment component (Marks et al. 1988). However, clomipramine doses in that study were rather low (i.e., 125–150 mg), and therapist-aided exposure was instituted late in the treatment and briefly. In a study comparing behavioral treatment with clomipramine treatment for children with OCD, the two treatments were similarly helpful, suggesting that non-pharmacological options might be a good first-line option in the younger population in an initial attempt to avoid medication (de Haan et al. 1998).

Cognitive and behavioral approaches to treating OCD are summarized in Table 7–4.

TABLE 7–4.   **Cognitive and behavioral approaches to treating obsessive-compulsive disorder**

Graded exposure (imaginal and/or in vivo)
Flooding
Response prevention
Cognitive restructuring

Cognitive Therapy

Cognitive therapy has also been advocated in the treatment of OCD, centering on cognitive reformulation of themes related to the perception of danger, estimation of catastrophe, expectations about anxiety and its consequences, excessive responsibility, thought-action fusion, and illogical inferences (Freeston et al. 1996; O'Connor and Robillard 1996; Rachman et al. 1995; vanOppen and Arntz 1994). A review of 15 open and controlled trials of cognitive therapy for OCD showed little evidence overall of improvement when cognitive therapy was added to existing pharmacological and behavioral techniques (James and Blackburn 1995). However, one controlled study showed cognitive therapy to have effectiveness similar to that of exposure and response prevention in treating OCD (vanOppen et al. 1995).

Other Psychotherapy

Patients with OCD frequently have symptoms that seem laden with unconscious symbolism and dynamic meaning. However, OCD has generally proven refractory to psychoanalytically oriented psychotherapies—as well as to loosely structured, nondirective, exploratory psychotherapies—and these have been largely abandoned as modalities for treating OCD. In contrast to its lack of efficacy in treating chronic OCD, dynamic psychotherapy may be helpful for dealing with acute and limited-symptom cases in patients who are otherwise psychologically minded and motivated to explore their conflicts. It is also effective in dealing with the obsessive character traits of perfectionism, doubting, procrastination, and indecisiveness (Salzman 1985). In addition, dynamic psychotherapy may be helpful in working through aspects of personality that feed into and further exacerbate the OCD symptoms or that affect broader interpersonal functioning above and beyond the OCD symptoms per se. However, controlled clinical data are not available to support these clinical impressions.

OCD patients need supportive treatment even while pharmacotherapy or behavioral therapy is being applied. Because of their tendency toward excessive doubt, these patients may require a great deal of reassurance during the early phase of treatment. More intensive supportive therapy that encourages risk taking helps OCD patients live with their anxiety, and a focus on the present has been reported to be helpful (Salzman 1985). In addition, educational support groups for OCD patients and their families have been described as highly successful in helping treat these patients (Black and Blum 1992; Tynes et al. 1992).

■ POSTTRAUMATIC STRESS DISORDER

General Psychotherapeutic Principles

It is generally agreed that some form of psychotherapy is necessary in the treatment of posttraumatic stress disorder (PTSD). Crisis intervention that takes place shortly after the traumatic event is effective in reducing immediate distress—possibly preventing chronic or delayed responses—and, if the pathological response is still tentative, may allow for briefer intervention. Brief dynamic psychotherapy has been advocated both as an immediate treatment procedure and as a way of preventing chronic disorder. In this brief dynamic psychotherapy, the therapist needs to establish an alliance that allows the patient to work through his or her reactions.

The literature has suggested that persons with disrupted early attachments or abuse, who have been traumatized earlier in their lives, are more likely to develop PTSD than those with stable backgrounds. The occurrence of psychic trauma in a person's past may psychologically and biologically predispose him or her to respond excessively and maladaptively to intense experiences and affects (Herman et al. 1989; Krystal 1968; van der Kolk 1987b). Therefore, attempting to modify preexisting conflicts, developmental difficulties, and defensive styles that render the person especially vulnerable to traumatization by particular experiences is central to the treatment of traumatic syndromes.

The phase-oriented treatment model suggested by Horowitz and colleagues (1976) strikes a balance between initial supportive interventions to minimize the traumatic state and increasingly aggressive "working through" at later stages of treatment. Establishing a safe and communicative relationship, reappraising the traumatic event, revising the patient's inner model of self and world, and working with the reexperiencing of loss activated by termination are all important therapeutic issues in the treatment of PTSD. Herman and her group (Herman et al. 1989) have emphasized the importance of validating the patient's traumatic experiences as a precondition for reparation of damaged self-identity.

Embry (1990) has outlined seven major parameters for effective psychotherapy with war veterans with chronic PTSD: 1) initial rapport building, 2) limit setting and supportive confrontation, 3) affective modeling, 4) defocusing on stress and focusing on current life events, 5) sensitivity to transference-countertransference issues, 6) understanding of secondary gain, and 7) maintaining a positive treatment attitude.

Group psychotherapy can also serve as an important adjunctive treatment or as the central treatment mode of traumatized patients (van der Kolk 1987a). Because of past experiences, such patients are often mistrustful and reluctant to depend on authority figures, whereas the identification, support, and hopefulness of peer settings can facilitate therapeutic change.

Medication treatment has been impressionistically reported to have a positive effect on psychotherapy in 70% of cases, with improvements in symptom severity leading to a more positive and motivated approach to psychotherapy and an enhancement of accessibility to uncovering and working through (Bleich et al. 1986).

Cognitive and Behavioral Therapies

A variety of cognitive and behavioral techniques have gained increasing popularity and validation in the treatment of PTSD. People involved in traumatic events frequently develop phobias or phobic anxiety related to or associated with these situations. When a phobic anxiety or avoidance is associated with PTSD, systematic desensitization or graded exposure has been found to be effective. This approach is based on the principle that when patients are gradually exposed to a phobic or anxiety-provoking stimulus they will become habituated or deconditioned to the stimulus. Variations of this treatment include using imaginal techniques (i.e., imaginal desensitization) and exposure to real-life situations, (i.e., in vivo desensitization). Prolonged exposure (i.e., flooding), if tolerated by a patient, can also be useful and has been reported to be successful in the treatment of a group of Vietnam War veterans (Fairbank and Keane 1982).

Relaxation techniques produce the beneficial physiological results of reducing motor tension and decreasing the activity of autonomic nervous system effects—results that may be particularly efficacious in PTSD. Progressive muscle relaxation technique involves contracting and relaxing various muscle groups to induce the relaxation response. This relaxation response is useful for symptoms of autonomic arousal such as somatic symptoms, anxiety, and insomnia. Hypnosis has also been used with success to induce the relaxation response in PTSD.

Cognitive therapy and *thought stopping*, in which a phrase and momentary pain are paired with thoughts or images of the trauma, have been used to treat unwanted mental activity in PTSD. A recent randomized trial compared imaginal exposure with cognitive therapy in 72 patients with chronic PTSD (Tarrier et al. 1999). Both treatments resulted in comparable major improvement—although not complete remission—of symptoms. Another controlled study of 87 patients with chronic PTSD compared exposure therapy, cognitive restructuring, their combination, and simple relaxation techniques (Marks et al. 1998). Both the behavioral treatment (exposure) and the cognitive treatment resulted in marked improvement, with gains maintained after 6 months, whereas the combination of the two treatments was of no additional benefit, and relaxation yielded modest improvement. In another study, exposure therapy, stress inoculation training, their combination, and a control waiting list were compared in assaulted women with chronic PTSD (Foa et al. 1999). All three active treatments resulted in comparable improvement, and the gains were maintained during up to 1 year of follow-up. In another study aiming to boost individual exposure therapy with family behavioral interventions, the latter rendered no additional benefit (Glynn et al. 1999).

Another approach, affect management, also appears to be beneficial. In a randomized study of adult women with PTSD and childhood sexual abuse who were already receiving individual psychotherapy and pharmacotherapy, those who underwent a 3-month course of group affect-management treatment demonstrated notably fewer PTSD symptoms and dissociative symptoms after the treatment (Zlotnick et al. 1997).

Affect management appears also to be highly beneficial for children and adolescents, although these pediatric patients have been less rigorously studied. In an open trial of CBT in 17 pediatric study subjects with PTSD, more than half no longer met disorder criteria after treatment and were doing even better at 6-month follow-up (March et al. 1998). Cognitive and behavioral techniques that can be useful in treating PTSD are summarized in Table 7–5.

TABLE 7–5.	**Cognitive and behavioral approaches to treating posttraumatic stress disorder**

Graded exposure (imaginal and/or in vivo)
Flooding
Progressive muscle relaxation
Hypnosis
Stress inoculation training
Cognitive restructuring
Thought stopping
Affect management

Other Treatments

Eye movement desensitization and reprocessing (EMDR) is a relatively new technique that has been applied to the treatment of trauma-related pathology in the past decade. There continues to be controversy in the literature regarding the efficacy of EMDR, as well as its underlying mechanisms of action. In a 5-year follow-up study of a small group of veterans who had initially been treated with EMDR with modest benefits, all benefit was lost at follow-up (Macklin et al. 2000). Although EMDR has been found to be superior to relaxation in treating PTSD (Carlson et al. 1998), the latter is not a top treatment of choice. A recent randomized study comparing EMDR with CBT found that the latter was notably more effective and its superiority even more apparent at 3-month follow-up (Devilly and Spence 1999).

■ REFERENCES

Agras S, Leitenberg H, Barlow DH: Social reinforcement in the modification of agoraphobia. Arch Gen Psychiatry 19:423–427, 1968

American Psychiatric Association: Diagnostic and Statistical Manual of Mental Disorders, 3rd Edition. Washington, DC, American Psychiatric Association, 1980

Arntz A, van den Hout M: Psychological treatments of panic disorder without agoraphobia: cognitive therapy versus applied relaxation. Behav Res Ther 34:113–121, 1996

Barlow DH, Craske MG, Cerny JA, et al: Behavioral treatment of panic disorder. Behav Ther 20:261–282, 1989

Barlow DH, Rapee RM, Brown TA: Behavioral treatment of generalized anxiety disorder. Behav Ther 23:551–570, 1992

Beck AT, Emery G, Greenberg RL: Anxiety Disorders and Phobias: A Cognitive Perspective. New York, Basic Books, 1985

Beck AT, Sokol L, Clark DA, et al: A crossover study of focused cognitive therapy for panic disorder. Am J Psychiatry 149:778–783, 1992

Beidel DC, Turner SM, Morris TL: Behavioral treatment of childhood social phobia. J Consult Clin Psychol 68:1072–1080, 2000

Black DW, Blum NS: Obsessive-compulsive disorder support groups: the Iowa model. Compr Psychiatry 33:65–71, 1992

Bleich A, Siegel B, Garb R, et al: Post-traumatic stress disorder following combat exposure: clinical features and psychopharmacological treatment. Br J Psychiatry 149:365–369, 1986

Borkovec TD, Costello E: Efficacy of applied relaxation and cognitive-behavioral therapy in the treatment of generalized anxiety disorder. J Consult Clin Psychol 61:611–619, 1993

Butler G, Fennell M, Robson P, et al: Comparison of behavior therapy and cognitive behavior therapy in the treatment of generalized anxiety disorder. J Consult Clin Psychol 59:167–175, 1991

Calvocoressi L, Lewis B, Harris M, et al: Family accommodation in obsessive-compulsive disorder. Am J Psychiatry 152:441–443, 1995

Carlson JG, Chemtob CM, Rusnak K, et al: Eye movement desensitization and reprocessing (EMDR) treatment for combat-related posttraumatic stress disorder. J Trauma Stress 11:3–24, 1998

Chambless DL, Gillis MM: Cognitive therapy of anxiety disorders. J Consult Clin Psychol 61:248–260, 1993

Clark DM: A cognitive model of panic attacks, in: Panic: Psychological Perspectives. Edited by Rachman S, Maser JD. Hillsdale, NJ, Erlbaum, 1988, pp 71–89

Cooper AM: Will neurobiology influence psychoanalysis? Am J Psychiatry 142:1395–1402, 1985

Cottraux J, Note I, Albuisson E, et al: Cognitive behavior therapy versus supportive therapy in social phobia: a randomized controlled trial. Psychother Psychosom 69:137–146, 2000

Craske MG, Brown TA, Barlow DH: Behavioral treatment of panic disorder: a two-year follow-up. Behav Ther 22:289–304, 1991

De Haan E, Hoogduin KA, Buitelaar JK, et al: Behavior therapy versus clomipramine for the treatment of obsessive-compulsive disorder in children and adolescents. J Am Acad Child Adolesc Psychiatry 37:1022–1029, 1998

Devilly GJ, Spence SH: The relative efficacy and treatment distress of EMDR and a cognitive-behavior trauma treatment protocol in the amelioration of posttraumatic stress disorder. J Anxiety Disord 13:131–157, 1999

Durham RC, Murphy R, Allan T, et al: Cognitive therapy, analytic psychotherapy and anxiety management training for generalized anxiety disorder. Br J Psychiatry 165:315–323, 1994

Embry CK: Psychotherapeutic interventions in chronic posttraumatic stress disorder, in Posttraumatic Stress Disorder: Etiology, Phenomenology, and Treatment. Edited by Wolf ME, Mosnaim AD. Washington, DC, American Psychiatric Press, 1990, pp 226–236

Fairbank TA, Keane TM: Flooding for combat-related stress disorders: assessment of anxiety reduction across traumatic memories. Behav Ther 13:499–510, 1982

Foa EB, Steketee G, Grayson JB, et al: Deliberate exposure and blocking of obsessive compulsive rituals: immediate and long-term effects. Behav Ther 15:450–472, 1984

Foa EB, Dancu CV, Hembree EA, et al: A comparison of exposure therapy, stress inoculation therapy, and their combination for reducing posttraumatic stress disorder in female assault victims. J Consult Clin Psychol 67:194–200, 1999

Franklin ME, Kozak MJ, Cashman L, et al: Cognitive-behavioral treatment of pediatric obsessive-compulsive disorder: an open clinical trial. J Am Acad Child Adolesc Psychiatry 37:412–419, 1998

Franklin ME, Abramowitz JS, Kozak MJ, et al: Effectiveness of exposure and ritual prevention for obsessive-compulsive disorder: randomized compared with nonrandomized samples. J Consult Clin Psychol 68:594–602, 2000

Freeston MH, Rheaume J, Ladouceur R: Correcting faulty appraisals of obsessional thoughts. Behav Res Ther 34:433–446, 1996

Gabbard GO: Psychodynamic Psychiatry in Clinical Practice. Washington, DC, American Psychiatric Press, 1990

Glynn SM, Eth S, Randolph ET, et al: A test of behavioral family therapy to augment exposure for combat-related posttraumatic stress disorder. J Consult Clin Psychol 67:243–251, 1999

Goldstein AJ, Chambless DL: A reanalysis of agoraphobia. Behav Ther 9:47–59, 1978

Heimberg RG, Dodge CS, Hope DA, et al: Cognitive behavioral group treatment for social phobia: comparison with a credible placebo control. Cognitive Therapy and Research 14:1–23, 1990

Herman JL, Perry JC, van der Kolk BA: Childhood trauma in borderline personality disorder. Am J Psychiatry 146:490–495, 1989

Horowitz MJ: Stress-Response Syndromes. New York, Jason Aronson, 1976

James IA, Blackburn IM: Cognitive therapy with obsessive-compulsive disorder. Br J Psychiatry 166:444–450, 1995

Keijsers GP, Hoogduin CA, Schaap CP: Predictors of treatment outcome in the behavioral treatment of obsessive-compulsive disorder. Br J Psychiatry 165:781–786, 1994

Krystal H: Massive Psychic Trauma. New York, International Universities Press, 1968

Lipsitz JD, Mannuzza S, Klein DF, et al: Specific phobia 10–16 years after treatment. Depress Anxiety 10:105–111, 1999

Macklin ML, Metzger LJ, Lasko NB, et al: Five-year follow-up study of eye movement desensitization and reprocessing therapy for combat-related posttraumatic stress disorder. Compr Psychiatry 41:24–27, 2000

March JS, Amaya-Jackson L, Murray MC, et al: Cognitive-behavioral psychotherapy for children and adolescents with posttraumatic stress disorder after a single-incident stressor. J Am Acad Child Adolesc Psychiatry 37:585–593, 1998

Marks I: Behavior therapy for obsessive-compulsive disorder: a decade of progress. Can J Psychiatry 42:1021–1027, 1997

Marks IM, Hodgson R, Rachman S: Treatment of chronic obsessive-compulsive neurosis by in vivo exposure: a two-year follow-up and issues in treatment. Br J Psychiatry 127:349–364, 1975

Marks IM, Lelliott P, Basoglu M, et al: Clomipramine, self-exposure and therapist-aided exposure for obsessive-compulsive rituals. Br J Psychiatry 152:522–534, 1988

Marks I, Lovell K, Noshirvani H, et al: Treatment of posttraumatic stress disorder by exposure and/or cognitive restructuring: a controlled study. Arch Gen Psychiatry 55:317–325, 1998

Mattick RP, Peters L, Clarke JC: Exposure and cognitive restructuring for social phobia: a controlled study. Behav Ther 20:3–23, 1989

McKay D: A maintenance program for obsessive-compulsive disorder using exposure with response prevention: 2-year follow-up. Behav Res Ther 35:367–369, 1997

Milrod B, Busch F, Leon AC, et al: Open trial of psychodynamic psychotherapy for panic disorder: a pilot study. Am J Psychiatry 157:1878–1880, 2000

Noyes R Jr, Reich JH, Christiansen J, et al: Outcome of panic disorder: relationship to diagnostic subtypes and comorbidity. Arch Gen Psychiatry 47:809–818, 1990

O'Connor K, Robillard S: Inference processes in obsessive-compulsive disorder: some clinical observations. Behav Res Ther 33:887–896, 1996

Ost LG, Breitholtz E: Applied relaxation versus cognitive therapy in the treatment of generalized anxiety disorder. Behav Res Ther 38:777–790, 2000

Ost LG, Westling BE: Applied relaxation vs cognitive behavior therapy in the treatment of panic disorder. Behav Res Ther 33:145–158, 1995

Rachman S, Thordarson DS, Shafran R, et al: Perceived responsibility: structure and significance. Behav Res Ther 33:779–784, 1995

Rice KM, Blanchard EB, Purcell M: Biofeedback treatments of generalized anxiety disorder: preliminary results. Biofeedback Self Regul 18:93–105, 1993

Salkovskis PM, Westbrook D: Behavior therapy and obsessional ruminations: can failure be turned into success? Behav Res Ther 27:149–160, 1989

Salkovskis PM, Jones DRO, Clark DM: Respiratory control in the treatment of panic attacks: replication and extension with concurrent measurement of behavior and pCO2. Br J Psychiatry 148:526–532, 1986

Salzman L: Comments on the psychological treatment of obsessive-compulsive patients, in Obsessive-Compulsive Disorder: Psychological and Pharmacological Treatment. Edited by Mavissakalian M, Turner SM, Michelson L. New York, Plenum, 1985, pp 155–165

Sanderson WC, Rapee RM, Barlow DH: The influence of an illusion of control on panic attacks induced via inhalation of 5.5% carbon dioxide-enriched air. Arch Gen Psychiatry 46:157–162, 1989

Shafran R, Ralph J, Tallis F: Obsessive-compulsive symptoms and the family. Bull Menninger Clinic 59:472–479, 1996

Sokol L, Beck AT, Greenberg RL, et al: Cognitive therapy of panic disorder: a nonpharmacological alternative. J Nerv Ment Dis 177:711–716, 1989

Spence SH, Donovan C, Brechman TM: The treatment of childhood social phobia: the effectiveness of a social skills training-based, cognitive-behavioral intervention, with and without parental involvement. J Child Psychol Psychiatry 41:713–762, 2000

Steketee GS, Foa EB, Grayson JB: Recent advances in the behavioral treatment of obsessive compulsives. Arch Gen Psychiatry 39:1365–1371, 1982

Tarrier N, Pilgrim H, Sommerfield C, et al: A randomized trial of cognitive therapy and imaginable exposure in the treatment of chronic posttraumatic stress disorder. J Consult Clin Psychol 67:13–18, 1999

Telch MJ, Lucas JA, Schmidt NB, et al: Group cognitive-behavioral treatment of panic disorder. Behav Res Ther 31:279–287, 1993

Turner SM, Beidel DC, Cooley-Quille MR: Two-year follow-up of social phobias treated with Social Effectiveness Therapy. Behav Res Ther 33:553–555, 1995

Tynes LL, Salin SC, Skiba W, et al: A psychoeducational and support group for obsessive-compulsive disorder patients and their significant others. Compr Psychiatry 33:197–201, 1992

van der Kolk BA: The role of the group in the origin and resolution of the trauma response, in Psychological Trauma. Edited by van der Kolk BA. Washington, DC, American Psychiatric Press, 1987a, pp 153–171

van der Kolk BA: The separation cry and the trauma response: developmental issues in the psychobiology of attachment and separation, in Psychological Trauma. Edited by van der Kolk BA. Washington, DC, American Psychiatric Press, 1987b, pp 31–62 vanOppen P, Arntz A: Cognitive therapy for obsessive-compulsive disorder. Behav Res Ther 32:79–87, 1994

vanOppen P, deHaan E, van Balkom AJ, et al: Cognitive therapy and exposure in vivo in the treatment of obsessive compulsive disorder. Behav Res Ther 33:379–390, 1995

Wiborg IM, Dahl AA: Does brief dynamic psychotherapy reduce the relapse rate of panic disorder? Arch Gen Psychiatry 53:689–694, 1996

Wlazlo Z, Schroeder-Hartwig K, Hand I, et al: Exposure in vivo vs social skills training for social phobia: long-term outcome and differential effects. Behav Res Ther 28:181–193, 1990

Woody SR, Chambless DL, Glass CR: Self-focused attention in the treatment of social phobia. Behav Res Ther 35:117–129, 1997

Zlotnick C, Shea TM, Rosen K, et al: An affect-management group for women with posttraumatic stress disorder and histories of childhood sexual abuse. J Trauma Stress 10:425–436, 1997

8

SELECTING AND
COMBINING TREATMENTS

Studies validating the use of combined treatments—versus psychopharmacological or psychotherapeutic monotherapies—for anxiety disorders are still relatively limited, compared with studies of each modality alone. However, the last decade in particular has seen a number of compelling studies in this area. Admittedly, studies that compare combined treatment with monotherapies are more challenging to conduct, for a number of reasons. They usually need to involve larger numbers of treatment cells and, therefore, bigger sample sizes. Also, they usually require the coming together of researchers who have expertise in various disciplines, who may traditionally not have engaged in much cross-talk with each other. Finally, they usually require a search for subjects who are both appropriate and willing to randomly undergo psychopharmacological treatment, psychotherapeutic treatment, or the two together. Regardless of research evidence, clinical wisdom often precedes rigorous experimental evidence, and many clinicians know that the combination of medication and some form of psychotherapy may yield the greatest long-term outcomes for many patients with anxiety disorders.

A number of issues pertain to whether a clinician should choose monotherapy (psychotherapy or pharmacotherapy) or combined therapy for a newly arrived patient seeking relief from an anxiety disorder. It is safe to say that studies to date have pretty well established, as a general rule, that cognitive-behavioral therapy (CBT) and pharmacotherapy have comparable efficacy in treating most anxiety disorders—possibly with the exception of specific phobia. It has also emerged as a general pattern, from studies to date, that medication treatment may have an edge when it comes to treating more severe symptoms or achieving more complete symptom remission, whereas CBT has the advantage when it comes to the longer-term maintenance of gains.

How does the clinician, then, decide which treatment to start with? One important issue in any clinical decision is patient choice. Patients often arrive with some notion, whether clearly formulated or only partly conscious, as to the type of treatment they would like to receive. For the most part, it behooves clinicians to respect that choice unless it is clearly contraindicated. A patient who wishes first to try psychotherapy—or medication—should generally have his or her wish respected, because both approaches are known to have at least some efficacy in anxiety disorders. It is also often the case that patients preselect the kind of clinician they see in consultation based on their preferences and biases. In these cases, it is important for the clinician not to allow his or her own biases or comfort with particular modalities to constrict the options available to the patient. Although there are exceptions to every guideline, good candidates for *medication monotherapy* are generally those with more severe or chronic symptoms, a positive bias toward medication, poor motivation for the use of cognitive-behavioral techniques, or limited interest in insight and working-through, or those who have tried psychotherapy and wish to try something new. Conversely, good candidates for initial *psychotherapy* are those who have an initial negative outlook toward the perceived stigmatizing effect or other adverse effects of medication, those with symptoms of somewhat lesser severity or more limited duration, those motivated to learn cognitive-behavioral techniques, those showing some initial curiosity or insight about what makes them "tick," and those who have not done well with pharmacotherapy alone.

When starting with any modality, it is of crucial importance to educate the patient from the start regarding all the treatment options and some of the advantages and disadvantages of each. Patients may not know that differing approaches can all be effective or may be unaware that combination treatments may offer greater gains for many patients than any kind of monotherapy alone. This educational approach sets the groundwork for future changes or additions to the course of treatment, and it helps keep patients from becoming demoralized if one treatment does not work, as well as helping clinicians save face in this event. For example, if an initial course of monotherapy of any type does not yield positive results, patients may be inclined to perceive the addition of another treatment or the switch from one to another as a failure; this feeling of failure is less likely to occur if the clinician has introduced from the start the notion of other types of treatment as very feasible possibilities. In another common scenario, a patient may get only partial results from one modality and sense the need for further gains. It is often more constructive, and accurate, for the clinician to frame this scenario as an opportunity to use additional modalities, rather than as a partial failure of the modality already attempted.

In yet another common scenario, patients may start to wonder about the mind-body dichotomy and question whether their initial perception—for example, that in their case the condition was more "psychological" or more "physical"—was accurate. Adequate information from the start can circumvent such pitfalls, helping to educate the patient that the mind and body interact in ways that are inseparable, and therefore any treatment that is effective for them is as good as any other. Sometimes, informing patients of research studies that clearly make this point—such as the landmark studies on obsessive-compulsive disorder (OCD) showing that effective CBT brings on brain changes similar to those brought about by effective medication—can have a very powerful positive impact.

It is also common for patients who are initially severely symptomatic to have limited capacity to use psychotherapeutic techniques, because their observing ego and their motivation to use helpful new cognitions and behaviors may be simply overwhelmed by their pathology. The clinician can again be very helpful to these patients by suggesting and explaining the sequencing of treatment in such cases. Medication will be expected to relieve symptoms enough to allow patients to further tackle them with psychotherapeutic approaches. In turn, these approaches may help patients in eventually discontinuing long-term medication, or using it only at times of exacerbation of their symptoms. All these concepts are supported by research and generally should be shared with patients from the start.

Finally, in another common scenario, patients may make enough gains in the treatment of their anxiety disorder, whether the treatment is psychopharmacological or psychotherapeutic, that they come to realize there are additional conflicts and life issues, such as associated character issues, that they would like to address and now have the "luxury" to do so. Having predicted this outcome, at least in cases in which it was reasonably obvious, can be very helpful in facilitating the introduction of later treatment interventions.

What about starting psychotherapy and pharmacotherapy concurrently with a new patient? The existing studies comparing combined treatment with monotherapy are summarized in this chapter. As a general conclusion, it can be said that the studies have often, but not always, found that combined treatment is better than monotherapy. Certainly, it is never worse. Therefore, with a new patient it might be overtreatment to start both treatments simultaneously, except in certain instances—for example, when patients are motivated from the start to try both and can invest the time, effort, and expense involved; when symptoms are severe and incapacitating and maximal results are needed quickly; or, of course, when patients have only partially responded already to one modality and are now coming to a clinician looking for further gains.

■ PANIC DISORDER

Compared to panic disorder with agoraphobia, less is known about the relative or combined efficacy of medications versus CBT in the treatment of panic disorder without agoraphobia. In one controlled study, fluvoxamine was notably beneficial in the acute treatment of panic disorder, whereas cognitive therapy did not surpass placebo (Black et al. 1993). On the contrary, another controlled study found cognitive therapy, relaxation, and imipramine to be similarly effective, and cognitive therapy had more lasting effects at 9 months follow-up after treatment was discontinued (Clark et al. 1994). After the initiation of medication treatment for initial symptom control, the introduction of CBT seems to greatly increase the likelihood that a patient will be able to successfully taper off medication (Otto et al. 1993).

Results from the largest study comparing medication, CBT, and combination therapy, acute and longer-term, were recently published (Barlow et al. 2000). The study was a multi-site controlled study of 312 patients with panic disorder, randomly assigned to five different treatments: imipramine alone, CBT alone, imipramine and CBT combined, placebo medication, and placebo plus CBT. In the initial 3-month acute treatment phase, medication and CBT independently had similar efficacy, with limited advantage to combined treatment with imipramine and CBT. For patients treated in the 6-month maintenance phase, imipramine produced a higher quality of response than CBT alone, and there was more substantial advantage than earlier with combined treatment. Finally, at 6-month follow-up after termination of treatment, CBT had more durable results. This study, the most comprehensive to date, clearly suggests that both psychotherapy and medication treatment must be seriously considered in treating a patient with panic disorder, each having its advantages and limitations.

There continues to be disagreement in the literature regarding the best method for treating panic disorder with agoraphobia. Antipanic medication is given to block the occurrence of panic attacks, and its efficacy in this regard is well documented. However, medication alone is often not adequate treatment for patients with significant agoraphobic avoidance. It is generally accepted that some means of exposing patients with agoraphobia to the feared situations is necessary for overall improvement. This exposure to the feared stimulus may be achieved by various nonspecific methods, such as education, reassurance, and supportive therapy (Klein et al. 1983). However, focused CBT is, on the whole, more successful than nonspecific techniques in reducing agoraphobic avoidance, as detailed in Chapter 7, "Psychotherapy Treatments." Consequently, the relative and combined efficacy of medications and CBT for panic disorder with agoraphobia has been the focus of a number of investigations.

Some studies have not found imipramine to have a significant effect on agoraphobia when given alone or with exposure instructions (Marks et al. 1983; Telch et al. 1985), whereas another study has shown imipramine alone to decrease phobic avoidance at combined plasma levels of 110–140 ng/mL (Mavissakalian and Perel 1995). Most studies concur that the combination of medication and behavioral treatment (exposure) are superior in treating phobic avoidance to medication or behavioral treatment alone (de Beurs et al. 1995; Mavissakalian and Michelson 1986; Telch et al. 1985; Zitrin et al. 1980).

In summary, antidepressants combined with CBT should generally be instituted in the treatment of panic disorder with agoraphobia. Combination therapy appears to be superior to either treatment alone. In a large controlled study of alprazolam plus exposure in patients with panic disorder with agoraphobia, improvements in panic attacks, in anticipatory anxiety, and in avoidance were found to be largely independent of each other, and only early improvement in avoidance predicted overall improvement after treatment (Basoglu et al. 1994). CBT has been shown to decrease panic attacks but not agoraphobia, whereas exposure reduces agoraphobia but not panic attacks (van den Hout et al. 1994).

■ GENERALIZED ANXIETY DISORDER

There are minimal data on the use of combined psychotherapy and medication in the treatment of generalized anxiety disorder (GAD). In one study comparing CBT alone, benzodiazepine alone, the two combined, and placebo (Power et al. 1990), CBT alone or with medication tended to emerge as superior. It appears, however, that the CBT component of the study was more intensive than the medication treatment, and further studies are clearly needed in this area.

■ SOCIAL PHOBIA

Combination treatment with CBT and medication for social phobia has received some attention. It appears that medication alone, compared with CBT alone, can have comparable results in the acute treatment of social phobia (Gelernter et al. 1991; Heimberg et al. 1998; Otto et al. 2000). In a rigorous comparison to phenelzine—the "gold standard" medication—cognitive-behavioral group therapy was essentially found to have similar efficacy at the end of a 12-week period, although it took a longer time to reach a response level and was inferior in some of the final measures (Heimberg et al. 1998). Furthermore, the question of the longer-term effect of the two forms of therapy is particularly relevant, because social phobia is a chronic condition. In a continuation of the previously described study (Heimberg et al. 1998), patients who were treatment responders continued treatment with phenelzine or CBT for a 6-month maintenance phase, and were then followed for an additional 6-month treatment-free phase (Liebowitz et al. 1999). Both treatments maintained their effectiveness for the first 6 months, with phenelzine preserving its slight superiority over CBT. However, after treatment ended, CBT was associated with a greater likelihood of maintaining a good response.

■ OBSESSIVE-COMPULSIVE DISORDER

Combination therapy is commonly used and recommended in the treatment of OCD. Unless symptoms are mild or the patient is highly motivated to start out with CBT techniques, a common approach used in clinical practice is to start with medication, to attain a degree of improvement that will allow better utilization of CBT, and then attempt to taper medication once CBT has been mastered and shown to be effective. In a recent study that tested this commonly used approach, it appeared quite effective. Patients who remained symptomatic with a 12-week course of a selective serotonin reuptake inhibitor (SSRI) were entered into a course of exposure and ritual prevention; they demonstrated a 50% decrease in their

OCD symptoms (Simpson et al. 1999). Another study compared behavioral or cognitive therapy alone to initial SSRI treatment later complemented with those therapies; the study showed no differences among these treatments. The findings were interpreted as suggesting that psychotherapy alone may be sufficient, at least in this group of subjects (van Balkom et al. 1998). Finally, a meta-analytic comparison study of OCD treatments, after controlling for a number of confounding variables, found that clomipramine, SSRIs, and exposure with response prevention have comparable results (Kobak et al. 1998).

■ POSTTRAUMATIC STRESS DISORDER

To our knowledge, there are as yet no studies published comparing pharmacological with psychological monotherapies, or examining the efficacy of combination treatments, in posttraumatic stress disorder (PTSD). Based on review and meta-analytic studies of each modality, pharmacotherapy and psychotherapy appear to have grossly comparable efficacy somewhere in the realm of 40%–70% (Davidson et al. 1997; Sherman 1998). Future studies are expected to shed more light on exact guidelines regarding these two approaches in PTSD.

■ EVALUATING RESPONSE TO TREATMENT

In order to make educated decisions regarding changes or additions in the modalities used to treat anxiety disorders, it is crucial to be able to do accurately appraise patients' progress. A generally useful strategy, as with assessing symptoms of any disorder in which the patient is a reasonably reliable rater, is to rate symptomatology at each visit so as to have simple quantifiable information that can be compared between visits. These ratings are best done without reminding patients of their previous ratings; sometimes patients will ask what their response was last time, and a response is best avoided. Some anxiety-ridden patients may have prohibitions from stating too much progress, such as the GAD patient whose worry can serve magical protective functions. Two easy questions to ask patients: 1) How much better are you now, percentage-wise, from when we first started treatment: 10%, 50%, 90%? and 2) If 0 is having no symptoms and 10 is the worst you have ever felt, how severe have your symptoms been, on average, in the past _____ [time period]? These ratings should, and typically do, complement closely the descriptive report that patients give of how they have been doing. If there is a major discrepancy between what patients describe and how they rate themselves, it should be clarified.

Another important principle in treating anxiety disorders is that avoidance is often present, and assessment of progress will not be accurate if, in addition to positive symptoms, avoidance is not closely monitored. For example, in panic disorder the clinician should inquire at each encounter about number and severity of panic attacks, presence of anticipatory anxiety, and presence of avoidance; the same 0–10 rating scale can be applied to each of the three components. A patient who is no longer having panic attacks, but whose agoraphobia remains the same, is clearly in need of further interventions. In contrast, anxiety patients may paradoxically appear more symptomatic and anxiety-ridden as they begin to make significant gains in confronting their avoidances. The increase in symptoms applies to GAD, social phobia, OCD, and PTSD.

In inquiring about GAD, it is useful to have compiled from the start a list of all of a patient's domains of worry and to be able to track the change in scope and intensity of each one, because sometimes new areas of worry can appear. In inquiring about social phobia, it is again important to ask about both anxiety and avoidance, because patients may not be experiencing the anxiety of social situations that are being totally avoided. It is also important to inquire about any change in the use of adjuvant measures, such as alcohol or necessary partners, that help deal with social situations.

In assessing change in OCD it is again useful to refer to an initial list of all then-present obsessions and compulsions and to inquire about them separately, because these may be multiple and change may vary among different symptoms. Also, the Yale-Brown Obsessive Compulsive Scale (Y-BOCS; Goodman et al. 1989) symptom checklist is very helpful for eliciting the various types of obsessions and compulsions. Useful questions to ask have to do with approximately how much time in the average day is taken up by symptoms, how able the patient is to resist the symptoms, and how successful the patient is at controlling them. The Y-BOCS severity scale may be helpful for quantifying the severity. Finally, with PTSD it is important to inquire about symptoms that may be present from all three domains—intrusive recollections, avoidance, and hyperarousal—because these may improve differentially with treatment.

As a last point, in the anxiety disorders as with all psychiatric disorders it is also crucial to assess not only improvement in anxiety symptoms, but also functional improvement regarding the range of activities that patients are able to engage in and the life satisfaction they are able to derive from the various aspects of their lives. If a person has demonstrated significant symptomatic improvement but remains disproportionately impaired, the clinician must wonder why and accordingly address this process. There are a number of possibilities that can be investigated. One is that the patient remains more symptomatic than meets the eye and that possibly there are some symptoms that have not been fully brought forth and credited for their seriousness. For example, some patients with OCD can sometimes show improvement in other areas but continue to hoard in ways that would seriously hamper any social life, if the hoarding precludes their ever inviting others to visit their home. Another possibility is that underlying personality disorder issues are preventing patients from attaining higher functioning, despite much symptomatic improvement. One example is the patient whose panic attacks have been fully treated, but who always finds reasons and excuses why a cognitive-behavioral program cannot be adhered to because it threatens the often-unconscious dependency on another person. A third possibility is that comorbid disorders are still leading to distress and dysfunction even though the anxiety disorder has been successfully treated, and those comorbid conditions should be addressed accordingly. For example, in any individual patient a medication that might be indicated for the treatment of both anxiety and depressive symptoms may work for one of the conditions but not for the other. Finally, some patients with anxiety disorders may have had so chronic a condition that they may have true deficits in their social or occupational capacities. In these situations, patients may greatly benefit from settings that will help teach them new social or vocational skills, such as group therapies or vocational programs.

■ REFERENCES

Barlow DH, Gorman JM, Shear MK, et al: Cognitive-behavioral therapy, imipramine, or their combination for panic disorder: a randomized controlled trial. JAMA 283:2529–2536, 2000

Basoglu M, Marks IM, Kilic C, et al: Relationship of panic, anticipatory anxiety, agoraphobia and global improvement in panic disorder with agoraphobia treated with alprazolam and exposure. Br J Psychiatry 164:647–652, 1994

Black DW, Wesner R, Bowers W, et al: A comparison of fluvoxamine, cognitive therapy, and placebo in the treatment of panic disorder. Arch Gen Psychiatry 50:44–50, 1993

Clark DM, Salkovskis PM, Hackmann A, et al: A comparison of cognitive therapy, applied relaxation therapy and imipramine in the treatment of panic disorder. Br J Psychiatry 164:759–769, 1994

Davidson JRT, Malik ML, Sutherland SN: Response characteristics to antidepressants and placebo in post-traumatic stress disorder. Review. Int Clin Psychopharmacol 12:291–296, 1997

de Beurs E, van Balkom AJ, Lange A, et al: Treatment of panic disorder with agoraphobia: comparison of fluvoxamine, placebo and psychological panic management combined with exposure and of exposure in vivo alone. Am J Psychiatry 152:683–691, 1995

Gelernter CS, Uhde TW, Cimbolic P, et al: Cognitive-behavioral and pharmacological treatments of social phobia: a controlled study. Arch Gen Psychiatry 48:938–945, 1991

Goodman WK, Price LH, Rasmussen SA, et al: The Yale-Brown Obsessive Scale I: development, use, and reliability. Arch Gen Psychiatry 46:1006–1011, 1989

Heimberg RG, Liebowitz MR, Hope DA, et al: Cognitive behavioral group therapy vs phenelzine therapy for social phobia: 12-week outcome. Arch Gen Psychiatry 55:1133–1141, 1998

Klein DF, Zitrin CM, Woerner MG, et al: Treatment of phobias, II: behavior therapy and supportive psychotherapy: are there any specific ingredients? Arch Gen Psychiatry 40:139–145, 1983

Kobak KA, Greist JH, Jefferson JW, et al: Behavioral versus pharmacological treatments of obsessive-compulsive disorder: a meta-analysis. Psychopharmacology (Berl) 136:205–216, 1998

Liebowitz MR, Heimberg RG, Schneier FR, et al: Cognitive-behavioral therapy versus phenelzine in social phobia: long-term outcome. Depress Anxiety 10:89–98, 1999

Marks IM, Gray S, Cohen D, et al: Imipramine and brief therapist-aided exposure in agoraphobics having self-exposure homework. Arch Gen Psychiatry 40:153–162, 1983

Mavissakalian M, Michelson L: Agoraphobia: relative and combined effectiveness of therapist-assisted in vivo exposure and imipramine. J Clin Psychiatry 47:117–122, 1986

Mavissakalian M, Perel JM: Imipramine treatment of panic disorder with agoraphobia: dose ranging and plasma level-response relationships. Am J Psychiatry 152:673–682, 1995

Otto MW, Pollack MH, Sachs GS, et al: Discontinuation of benzodiazepine treatment: efficacy of cognitive-behavioral therapy for patients with panic disorder. Am J Psychiatry 150:1485–1490, 1993

Otto MW, Pollack MH, Gould RA, et al: A comparison of the efficacy of clonazepam and cognitive-behavioral group therapy for the treatment of social phobia. J Anxiety Disord 14:345–358, 2000

Power KG, Simpson RJ, Swanson V, et al: A controlled comparison of cognitive-behavior therapy, diazepam, and placebo, alone and in combination, for the treatment of generalized anxiety disorder. J Anxiety Disord 4:267–292, 1990

Sherman JJ: Effects of psychotherapeutic treatments for PTSD: a meta-analysis of controlled clinical trials. J Trauma Stress 11:413–435, 1998

Simpson HB, Gorfinkle KS, Liebowitz MR: Cognitive-behavioral therapy as an adjunct to serotonin reuptake inhibitors in obsessive-compulsive disorder: an open trial. J Clin Psychiatry 60:584–590, 1999

Telch MJ, Agras WG, Taylor CM, et al: Combined pharmacological and behavioral treatment for agoraphobia. Behav Res Ther 23:325–335, 1985 van Balkom AJ, de Haan E, van Oppen P, et al: Cognitive and behavioral therapies alone versus in combination with fluvoxamine in the treatment of obsessive-compulsive disorder. J Nerv Ment Dis 186:492–499, 1998

van den Hout M, Arntz A, Hoekstra R: Exposure reduced agoraphobia but not panic, and cognitive therapy reduced panic but not agoraphobia. Behav Res Ther 32:447–451, 1994

Zitrin CM, Klein DF, Woerner MG: Treatment of agoraphobia with group exposure in vivo and imipramine. Arch Gen Psychiatry 37:63–72, 1980

INDEX

*Page numbers printed in **boldface** type refer to tables or figures.*